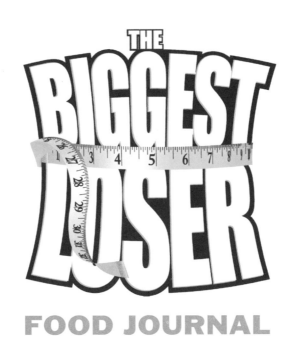

FOOD JOURNAL

The Biggest Loser Experts and Cast

RODALE

Rodale books may be purchased for business or promotional use or for special sales. For information, please write to: Special Markets Department, Rodale Inc., 733 Third Avenue, New York, NY 10017.

Printed in the United States of America
Rodale Inc. makes every effort to use acid-free ♾, recycled paper ♺.

Book design by Christina Gaugler

Illustration on page 5 by Judy Newhouse
Recipe photographs by Mitch Mandel/Rodale Images, except for those on pages 75 and 141, which are by John Yohman. All other photos by NBC Photo.

Library of Congress Cataloging-in-Publication Data

The biggest loser food journal / by The Biggest Loser Experts and Cast.
        p.   cm.
Includes index.
ISBN-13 978–1–60529–216–8   paperback
ISBN-10 1–60529–216–8   paperback
1. Reducing diets.   I. Biggest loser (Television program)
RM222.2.B533 2010
613.2'5—dc22   2010014295

Distributed to the trade by Macmillan
6   8   10   9   7   5   paperback

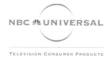

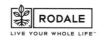

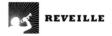

We inspire and enable people to improve their lives and the world around them.

INTRODUCTION

Year after year, you've watched the contestants on *The Biggest Loser* dramatically change their lives by losing weight and getting healthy. It's no secret that amenities such as a 24-hour gym, world-class trainers, a team of medical and nutrition experts, and a kitchen stocked with healthy foods give *The Biggest Losers* an edge on weight loss. But if you ask any contestant, past or present, to name the most valuable tool in his or her weight-loss journey, you'll hear the same answer: a food journal.

Keeping a food journal is something *The Biggest Losers* are required to do at the Ranch, and it quickly becomes a healthy habit they maintain for life. Why is a food journal so important? There are two main reasons. First, writing down everything you eat helps you understand exactly what foods, and how many calories, you're putting in your body—so if you lose, gain, or plateau from one week to the next, you have a written record of how you got there, and you can plan for the results you want. Second, tracking every meal, snack, and beverage you consume keeps you honest about all those little tastes and nibbles that occur throughout the day and makes you accountable for the results. As Season 8's Abby Rike says, "Accountability is key to losing weight. Keeping a food journal ensures that I'm aware of what I'm eating. I make sure I know how many calories I consume each day."

If you're not accountable for what you're eating, you won't lose weight. It is imperative to keep track of the number of calories you take in (and burn off through exercise) each day, especially when you're just getting started. Writing down what you eat will also help you identify which foods work for you and which foods don't. And, perhaps most important, knowing that you have to record every morsel you put in your mouth will make you think twice before mindlessly munching on foods that can undermine your weight-loss efforts! As Season 2's Jeff Levine says, "Before you put something in your mouth, ask yourself, 'Am I hungry?' Recognize your specific food and eating triggers and develop strategies to modify, limit, or avoid them."

Need more evidence that a food journal is essential to weight loss? How about this: A 2008 study conducted by Kaiser Permanente's Center for Health Research found that people who kept a food journal lost *twice* as much weight as those who relied on dieting and exercising alone!

In this daily food journal, you'll find pages for setting goals, recording your meals and snacks, and logging workouts. All three of these components—setting goals, tracking calories, and exercising—are crucial for weight loss. In the pages that follow, you'll learn more about *The Biggest Loser* food plan and how to calculate your daily calorie budget. You'll also find delicious recipes, exercise pointers, and tips from *The Biggest Loser* experts and cast.

Whether you're just starting out or have been following *The Biggest Loser* plan for a while, this tool will help you stay on track and achieve your goals. So let's get started. Begin journaling—and losing—today!

THE BIGGEST LOSER PLAN

WHAT IS A CALORIE?

A calorie is a measurement of how much energy the food you eat provides for your body. You need energy to fuel physical activity as well as all metabolic processes, from maintaining your heartbeat to healing a broken bone or building lean muscle mass. Only four components of the food you eat supply calories: protein and carbohydrates (4 calories per gram), alcohol (7 calories per gram), and fat (9 calories per gram). Vitamins, minerals, fiber, and water do not supply calories.

Keep in mind that the quality of your calories is just as important as the quantity. Some calories will fuel your workouts, keep you feeling full and satisfied, and help boost your body's immune system and protect you from disease. Other calories (often referred to as "empty calories") don't really provide any benefits—in fact, they can make you feel tired, sluggish, and hungrier than you were before you ate. *The Biggest Loser* plan will show you how to fuel your body the right way. When you give your body the nutrients and energy it needs, you will not only lose weight, you'll also feel better than ever.

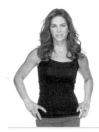

The Biggest Loser plan helps you determine the exact daily calorie intake you require to meet your individual weight-loss goals. If you weigh 150 pounds or more, the simple calorie budget formula on page 2, created by

Biggest Loser Trainer Tip: Jillian Michaels

Let go of the word *diet* and build a lifestyle that fits you. The key to success is balance.

The Biggest Loser experts, will help you calculate how many calories you need each day. If you weigh less than 150 pounds, talk to your doctor about a calorie budget based on your individual weight-loss needs.

Calorie Budget Calculation

Your present weight × 7 = your daily calorie need for weight loss

As you lose weight, you'll need to reassess and reduce your calorie budget continually in order to break through plateaus and keep losing weight. As you know from watching the show, *The Biggest Loser* contestants lose a lot of weight during their first few weeks at the Ranch. But after they've been at the Ranch for a while and have less weight to lose, they must increase the intensity of their workouts and carefully track their calories to keep losing.

Age is another factor in weight loss. Our muscles burn a lot of calories each day—about 10 times as many as our fat tissue does. Muscles shrink with age, however, which means we have a natural tendency to burn fewer calories as we get older. So, as our muscle decreases, our body fat increases. While you may lose weight more slowly as you get older, don't let that hold you back from your goals. Season 7's Helen Phillips became *The Biggest Loser* at the age of 48, beating much younger contestants for the grand prize. She's living proof that you can get healthy at any age!

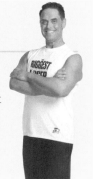

Michael Ventrella, Season 9 Winner

Each day you are going to feel better than the one before. You will move better, you will not be as tired, and you will enjoy a little more of each day. Strive to do more and be better than who you were yesterday.

ALLOCATING YOUR CALORIES

Now that you've determined your daily calorie budget, the next step is to figure out how many calories to allocate for each meal and snack. On *The Biggest Loser* plan, you'll eat three meals and two snacks a day.

Divide your total daily calorie budget by four to determine how many calories you should spend on each meal and snack. The example below uses a sample calorie budget of 1,800—yours may be more or less, depending on your goal and starting weight.

Total daily calorie budget: 1,800

$$1,800 \div 4 = 450$$

So for each meal—breakfast, lunch, and dinner—this person has a 450-calorie budget.

Now divide the remaining one-fourth of your total daily calorie budget—in this case, 450—by two.

$$450 \div 2 = 225$$

So for each of two daily snacks, this person has a 225-calorie budget.

This equation is just a starting point. Use it to help you determine a distribution of calories throughout the day that keeps you satisfied. If you go to the gym in the morning, for example, and require a bigger breakfast to fuel your workout, feel free to shift your calorie intake toward the start of your day. You can move your calorie distribution around to suit your needs and schedule.

If you prefer to eat several small meals a day, you can do that, too. Six 300-calorie meals throughout the day is certainly an option for someone on an 1,800-calorie budget. But as Season 7's Blaine Cotter says, "There's something so satisfying about that feeling of fullness that follows a regular meal. I would miss it too much if I only had small meals!"

In order to gauge the calorie content of your meals and snacks accurately, you'll need to familiarize yourself with serving sizes. It's important to weigh and measure food so that you know exactly how many calories you're consuming. It's useful to have the following tools (many of which you may already own) to help you measure your portion sizes.

- Liquid measuring cup (2-cup capacity)
- Set of dry measuring cups (includes 1-cup, ½-cup, ⅓-cup, and ¼-cup sizes)
- Measuring spoons (1 tablespoon, 1 teaspoon, ½ teaspoon, and ¼ teaspoon)
- The Biggest Loser Food Scale
- Calculator

Be sure that your food scale measures grams. (A gram is very small, about 1/28 of an ounce.) Most of your weight measurements will be in ounces, but certain foods, such as nuts, are very concentrated in calories, so you may need to measure your portion sizes of those foods in grams. There are a wide range of food scales available these days. To purchase the same scale the contestants use at the Ranch, go to biggestloser.com.

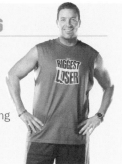

Brady Vilcan, Season 6

Buy a food scale. Portion size can get away from you in a heartbeat. If you want to lose weight, you have to know what a serving is and how many calories are in it.

A calculator will be indispensable for tallying your calories at the end of the day. It can also come in handy when the portion size of a food you want to eat differs from the suggested serving listed on its packaging—you may have to do a little math to figure out how many calories you're actually consuming.

When you're making your meals at home, weigh and measure your food *after* cooking. A food's weight can change dramatically when cooked. For example, 4 ounces of boneless, skinless chicken breast has around 130 calories when raw. When it's cooked, it'll weigh closer to 3 ounces but will have nearly the same calorie content. The same holds true for vegetables and other cooked foods. Dry cereals or grains, on the other hand, can double or even triple in volume after being cooked with water. Remember that an ounce of weight is not the same as a fluid ounce. You cannot convert the two without knowing the density of the ingredient you're measuring.

After precisely measuring your foods for a week or so, you'll be able to make fairly accurate estimates on your own. Over time, you'll know what right-size portions look like, whether you're cooking a meal in your own kitchen or deciding how much of your entrée to eat in a restaurant (and how much of it to wrap up and take home). But in the beginning, the tools mentioned above can help you get it just right. You can refer to the conversion table on page 244 of the Appendix for a list of common measurements and conversions. It can be helpful to refer to this chart when you're dining out or cooking a meal at home.

THE BIGGEST LOSER PLAN

The Biggest Loser nutrition pyramid is made up of fruits and vegetables at its base, protein foods on the second tier, and whole grains on the third tier. The top tier is a 200-calorie budget for healthy fats and "extras."

On *The Biggest Loser* 4-3-2-1 plan, you will eat a daily minimum of four servings of fruits and vegetables; up to three servings of healthy protein; up to two servings of whole grains; and up to one serving of "extras."

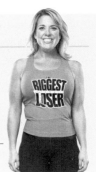

Abby Rike, Season 8

When eating out, decide what you're in the mood for. Then make modifications to the menu that's available to you. Be specific about how you want your food prepared— it can make a big difference.

THE 4-3-2-1 *BIGGEST LOSER* PYRAMID

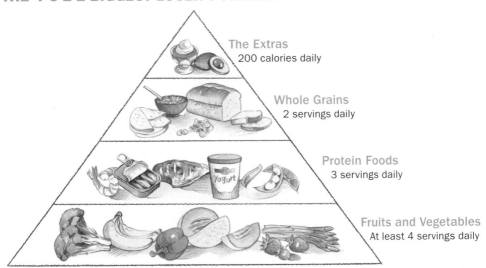

The Extras
200 calories daily

Whole Grains
2 servings daily

Protein Foods
3 servings daily

Fruits and Vegetables
At least 4 servings daily

45 Percent of Your Daily Calories: Vegetables, Fruit, and Whole Grains

At the base of the pyramid, fruits and vegetables supply most of your daily nutrients in the form of vitamins, minerals, and fiber and contain relatively low numbers of calories. Aim for a minimum of 4 cups of a variety of fruits and nonstarchy vegetables daily. You can eat more than four servings a day of most fruits and vegetables if you wish, though the majority of your choices should be vegetables.

Vegetables: Serving size = 1 cup or 8 ounces

Tips for Eating Vegetables

- When cooking vegetables, avoid added fat; steam, grill, or stir-fry veggies in a nonstick skillet with a spray (not a splash) of healthy oil.
- Try to eat at least one vegetable raw each day. Try a new vegetable each week so that you don't get bored.
- Eat a vegetable salad for lunch or dinner most days of the week.
- Keep precut vegetables such as bell peppers, celery, broccoli, and jicama in your fridge for easy snacking at home or to take to work or school.
- Starchier vegetables such as pumpkin, winter squash, and sweet potatoes are higher in calories and carbs, so limit them to one or two servings per week.
- Fresh vegetables are best, but you can choose frozen as well. If you opt for canned, be sure to rinse the contents before eating to wash away added salt.

Fruit: Serving size = 1 cup, 1 medium piece, or 8 ounces

Tips for Eating Fruit

- Enjoy at least one whole fruit each day. Apples, oranges, pears, bananas, and grapes are all easily portable and can be eaten for snacks on the go.
- Dark green, light green, orange, purple, red, and yellow: Savor fruits from different color groups. This ensures that you're getting a variety of nutrients.

- Eat fruit for dessert! Many *Biggest Losers* who have a sweet tooth use this strategy to curb their cravings.

- Opt for fresh fruit over dried fruit, which is more concentrated in calories and sugar and less filling.

- Choose whole fruit rather than fruit juices. Fruit juice contains less fiber, so it's not as filling as whole fruit, and it's more concentrated in sugars, so it will cause a greater spike in your blood sugar. When you do choose juice, keep in mind that a serving size is 4 ounces (½ cup).

- Fresh fruit is preferable, but frozen fruit is fine as long as it's not packaged with added sugar or syrup. If you choose canned fruit, be sure it's packed in water.

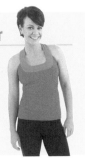

Whole Grains: Serving size = 1 cup of cooked grains or 2 slices of bread

Choose whole grain foods in moderation and select those with high fiber content. On *The Biggest Loser* plan, you'll eat two servings of whole grains daily. When grains are refined, important nutrients are removed. All that's usually left is starch, which is loaded with carbohydrate calories and little else. *Whole grains* undergo minimal processing and thus retain most of their nutritional value. The whole grain family includes barley, corn, oats, quinoa, rice, and wheat. These are all great sources of protein,

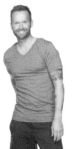

B vitamins, antioxidants, and fiber. On page 245 of the Appendix, you'll find a chart that lists the fiber content of many common whole grains.

Tips for Eating Whole Grains

- When choosing bread products, read the label carefully. If it says "enriched," the product probably contains white flour—meaning it's low in fiber and nutrition.

- Choose breads with at least 2 grams of fiber per serving, but aim for 5 grams. When you read the ingredient list, look for "whole wheat" or "whole grain" among the first few ingredients. "Wheat flour" isn't necessarily whole wheat.

- Most packaged breakfast cereals are highly processed and loaded with added sugar. Choose cereals with fewer than 5 grams of sugar and at least 5 grams of fiber per serving.

- White flour, white sugar, white bread, and packaged baked goods affect your blood sugar and insulin too quickly—you don't want an excess of either in your bloodstream. And unlike their whole grain counterparts, these foods also lack antioxidants and fiber. Choose whole grains that will keep you feeling fuller, longer.

30 Percent of Your Daily Calories: Protein

Protein is a macronutrient found in meat, fish, poultry, eggs, and dairy products and in smaller amounts in beans, nuts, and whole grains. Protein is required to build and repair muscle, skin, hair, blood vessels, and other bodily tissues. Generally speaking, any food containing at least 9 grams of protein per serving is a high-protein food.

Lean proteins contain valuable nutrients that can help you achieve a healthy weight. Include protein in each meal and each snack so your body can benefit from it all day long. When you haven't eaten enough protein, you might find yourself running low on energy or suffering from muscle fatigue. Try to eat a little bit of protein or drink a protein shake within 30 minutes after a workout to help your muscles repair. In addition to helping to build muscle, protein also promotes the feeling of satiety, or fullness, thus curbing your appetite and keeping you from consuming extra calories. When combined with a carbohydrate (such as a piece of fruit), protein helps slow the release of blood sugar, sustaining your energy for longer periods of time.

Choose a variety of proteins to make up your three daily servings. Try to limit consumption of lean red meat to twice a week and avoid processed meats, such as bologna, hot dogs, and sausage, which are typically high in sodium and contain nitrates.

To figure out how many grams of protein should constitute each of your three daily servings, apply the formula below, which uses an 1,800-calorie budget as an example.

$$1,800 \times 0.30 = 540 \text{ calories from protein}$$

Then convert the calories to grams.

$$540 \div 4 \text{ calories per gram} = 135 \text{ grams of protein}$$

You can then allocate protein goals for each meal and snack, based on your total daily protein intake. Using the example above, daily protein servings might look like this:

Breakfast: 33 grams

Snack 1: 17 grams

Lunch: 34 grams

Snack 2: 17 grams

Dinner: 34 grams

Animal Protein: Serving size = 1 cup or 8 ounces

Meat

Choose lean cuts of meat, such as pork tenderloin and beef round, chuck, sirloin, or tenderloin. USDA Choice or USDA Select grades of beef usually have lower fat content. Avoid meat that is heavily marbled and remove any visible fat. Try to find ground meat that is at least 95 percent lean.

Poultry

The leanest poultry is the skinless white meat from the breast of chicken or turkey. When purchasing ground chicken or turkey, ask for the white meat.

Seafood

Seafood is an excellent source of protein, omega-3 fatty acids, vitamin E, and selenium. When you're buying seafood, go for options that are rich in omega-3 fatty acids, such as herring, mackerel, salmon, sardines (water packed), trout, and tuna.

Dairy: Serving size = 1 cup or 8 ounces

Top choices include fat-free (skim) milk, 1% (low-fat) milk, buttermilk, plain fat-free or low-fat yogurt, fat-free or low-fat yogurt with fruit (no sugar added), fat-free or low-fat cottage cheese, and fat-free or low-fat ricotta cheese. Light soy milks and soy yogurts are also fine, but if you eat soy because of a dairy intolerance or allergy, be sure to select soy products that are fortified with calcium. Egg whites are another excellent source of fat-free protein.

If you're not eating three servings of dairy per day, *The Biggest Loser* nutrition team recommends that you consider taking a calcium supplement.

Vegetarian Protein: Serving size = 1 cup or 8 ounces

Good sources of vegetarian protein include beans, nuts and seeds, and traditional soy foods, such as tofu and edamame. Many of these foods are also loaded with fiber.

25 Percent of Your Daily Calories: Good Fats

Healthy fats play a role in weight loss because they help you feel full and satisfied. But remember: Even good fats are a concentrated source of calories, and as such, you need to monitor your serving sizes carefully. Many of your calories from fat will be hidden in your carbohydrate and protein food choices. You'll have a small budget of leftover calories to spend on healthy fat and "extras."

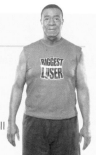

Mo DeWalt, Season 8

Down south, we deep-fry our fish. It tastes great, but it's horrible for your arteries. That same fish can be baked with seasonings. Try salmon with dill or flounder with lemon pepper.

Fats should make up no more than 25 percent of your total daily calories, and saturated fats should account for no more than 10 percent of your daily calorie budget. Here's how to calculate your daily fat intake, again based on the example of an 1,800-calorie budget.

Multiply your total daily calorie budget by 0.25 to see how many calories can come from fat.

$$1,800 \times 0.25 = 450$$

So up to 450 of this person's daily calories may come from fat.

One gram of fat contains 9 calories. So simply divide the number of calories from fat that you're allotted each day (in this case, 450) by nine.

$$450 \div 9 = 50$$

A person with an 1,800-calorie budget would consume no more than 50 grams of fat daily.

Tips for Eating Healthy Fats

- Choose olive oil, canola oil, flaxseed oil, or walnut oil for salads, cooking, and baking.
- When adding fat to a sandwich, try using reduced-fat mayonnaise or a little mashed avocado.
- Snack on nuts and seeds in moderation. Nut butters, trail mix, and raw nuts pack a powerful energy punch and supply a good dose of unsaturated fat. Keep portion sizes moderate; for example, 14 walnut halves make a 1-ounce serving.
    - Choose unsaturated fats. Many unsaturated fats, classified as monounsaturated or polyunsaturated, can lower your LDL (bad) cholesterol and raise your HDL (good) cholesterol.
    - Avoid trans fat, which is artificial fat found in hard margarines and vegetable shortenings, packaged baked goods, and foods fried in hydrogenated

Biggest Loser Trainer Tip: Bob Harper

Olive oil is not a source of empty calories—it's good for you. It may be high in calories, but in moderation, it is a heart-healthy option.

fats. Carefully read labels of packaged foods. If you see the words "hydrogenated" or "partially hydrogenated," put the package back on the shelf.

DECODING FOOD PACKAGING

Keeping a food journal will require you to become an expert at reading food labels and Nutrition Facts panels. When you're shopping for healthy foods, labels can help you choose between similar products based on calorie and nutrient (such as fat, protein, or fiber) content.

The label on this page is an example of what you'll find on the packaging of any item at your local supermarket. It contains a lot of information, but here is a list of what you most need to evaluate to make healthy choices.

Serving size: Everything else on the label (calories, grams of fat, etc.) is based on this measurement. Just because a food label suggests a certain portion doesn't mean that it's the right serving size for you. Look at the calorie and fat content that corresponds to the serving size. If you need to, cut the serving size in half. Also, be sure to check serving size on small items that you assume are one serving—often, they contain two or more servings per package.

Calories: This lists calories per serving. Be sure that the number of calories you record in your food journal reflects the number of calories you've eaten. If the label indicates that a serving is 1 cup and you ate 2 cups, you need to double the per-serving calorie number in order to record your double serving in your journal.

Total fat: The number of grams of fat in a product reflects the sum of three kinds of fat: saturated fat, polyunsaturated fat, and monounsaturated fat. Pay special attention to the

Nutrition Facts

Serving Size
Servings Per Container

Amount Per Serving

Calories 0

Calories from Fat 0

	% Daily Value*
Total Fat 0g	0%
Saturated Fat 0g	0%
Trans Fat 0g	
Cholesterol 0mg	0%
Sodium 0mg	0%
Total Carbohydrate 0g	0%
Dietary Fiber 0g	0%
Soluble Fiber 0g	0%
Insoluble Fiber 0g	0%
Sugars 0g	
Protein 0g	

Vitamin A 0%	·	Vitamin C 0%
Calcium 0%	·	Iron 0%
Phosphorus 0%	·	Magnesium 0%

* Percent Daily Values are based on a 2,000 calo-rie diet. Your daily values may be higher or lower depending on your calorie needs:

		Calories:	2,000	2,500
Total Fat	Less than		0g	0g
Sat Fat	Less than		0g	0g
Cholesterol	Less than		0mg	0mg
Sodium	Less than		0mg	0mg
Potassium			0mg	0mg
Total Carbohydrate			0g	0g
Dietary Fiber			0g	0g

Calories per gram:
Fat 0 · Carbohydrate 0 · Protein 0

INGREDIENTS: Whole Wheat Flour, (Stone Ground Whole Oats, Hard Red Winter Wheat, Rye, Long Grain Brown Rice, Triticale, Buckwheat, Barley, Sesame Seeds), Malted Barley, Salt, Yeast, Mixed Tocopherols (Natural Vitamin E) for Freshness.

numbers of calories in "light," reduced-fat, low-fat, and fat-free products. When the fat is removed from many recipes, salt or sugar is sometimes added to enhance the flavor. This can result in a fat-free or low-fat product that actually contains more calories than the regular version.

Saturated fat: Less than one-third of your daily grams of fat should come from saturated fats, which are derived mainly from animal products and are solid at room temperature (such as butter and shortening). Some plant oils, such as coconut oil and palm oil, also contain saturated fats. The saturated fat from animal foods is the primary source of cholesterol.

Sodium: For most people, the daily recommended sodium intake is no more than 2,400 milligrams. Some of the foods you eat each day will have more sodium than others. Aim for an average of no more than 240 milligrams of sodium in each meal or snack.

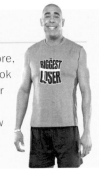

Allen Smith, Season 8

When you're at the grocery store, pay attention to the labels. Look at what you're putting into your body. Just because it says "low fat" doesn't mean it's low in calories. You have to count those calories!

Total carbohydrate: This number is calculated by adding grams of complex carbohydrates plus grams of fiber plus grams of sugars. Try to select carbohydrate foods with less than 10 grams of carbohydrate for each gram of fiber. For example, if a serving has 3 grams of fiber, it should have no more than 30 grams total of carbohydrate. Otherwise it is too refined or processed.

Dietary fiber: Fiber is found in plant foods but not in animal foods. Unless you're on a fiber-restricted diet, aim for at least 25 to 35 grams of fiber per day.

Sugars: The sugars in a food can be naturally occurring or added. Check the ingredient list to find out, and avoid eating foods that contain processed sugars, such as high-fructose corn syrup. The total grams of carbohydrates in a food serving should be more than twice the number of grams of sugars.

Protein: If a food has more than 9 grams of protein per serving, it's considered a high-protein food. It's important to eat foods that are high in protein when you're trying to lose weight, because protein is a great source of energy and helps you feel full.

Ingredient list: A product's ingredients are listed in order of decreasing weight. If the first few

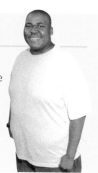

ingredients listed include any form of sugar (including cane sugar, corn syrup, sucrose, and so on) or fats and oils, the food is probably not a good choice for weight loss. Also, look for products with a short list of ingredients you recognize. A long list of strange-sounding ingredients is always a red flag.

STRUCTURING YOUR DAY

As you already know, on *The Biggest Loser* plan, you'll eat three meals (breakfast, lunch, and dinner) and two snacks a day. Parceling out your calories throughout the day means you'll stay full and won't go on sugar or carb binges to satisfy your growling stomach. It also means you won't go to bed feeling stuffed and sick from too many bad, empty calories. Ed Brantley of Season 6, a professional chef, used to eat his first meal of the day at lunchtime, when he'd scarf down a few burgers. It started a cycle of bad choices that continued throughout the day.

Eating more-frequent meals and snacks will . . .

- Keep you from feeling deprived.
- Help control blood sugar and insulin levels. (Insulin is a fat-forming hormone.)
- Lead to lower body fat.
- Keep you energized for exercise and activity.
- Reduce stress hormones in the body that can contribute to fat accumulation.
- Establish a regular pattern of eating that helps prevent impulse eating.

"At first, I really had to work to get all my meals in," recalls Danny Cahill, the Season 8 winner. "I wasn't used to eating healthy. I quickly realized that nutrient-dense foods were more satisfying than all the fat I was getting from fast food. It kept up my energy level, and I felt fueled for workouts."

Contestants are often surprised to learn that their past habit of skipping meals contributed to their weight gain. One problem with skipping meals is that by the time mealtime rolls around, you're famished and more likely to choose the wrong foods, especially those high in fat. Fat has more than twice as many calories as protein and carbohydrate. It satisfies hunger very quickly, and your body seems to know this. So the longer you go without food, the more likely you are to crave a high-fat treat.

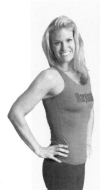 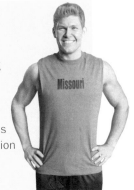

Amy and Marty Wolff, Season 3

When it comes to planning our dinner, we don't necessarily think about what we *want* to have— we plan for what our bodies *need*. That takes the emotion away and focuses us on nurturing our bodies.

Another problem with skipping meals is that when you wait too long to eat, you lose sight of your body's natural hunger cues. You don't really know when you're hungry anymore, or when you're full. Most overeaters don't stop eating when they're full—they stop when they're stuffed!

From starving to stuffed, the hunger scale on page 16 defines your body's hunger signals and how to interpret them.

If your hunger is anywhere from level 1 through 3, you should eat.

If you're at level 4, drink a glass of water, chew a piece of sugar-free gum, or do something else to distract yourself from thinking about food.

When you're trying to lose weight, you should try to stop eating when

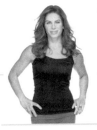

Biggest Loser Trainer Tip: Jillian Michaels

Losing weight is not about starving yourself; it's about eating what you want with certain modifications.

Hunger Scale

1. Famished or starving; you actually feel weak or light-headed. Don't allow yourself to get to this point.

2. Very hungry; you can't think of anything else but eating. You're cranky and irritable, and you can't concentrate.

3. Hungry; your stomach is growling or feels empty.

4. A little bit hungry; you're just starting to think about your next meal.

5. Satisfied; you're comfortable and aren't really thinking about food. You're alert and have a good energy level.

6. Fully satisfied; you've had enough to eat.

7. More than satisfied; you've had plenty to eat—maybe a little too much. Maybe you took a few extra bites.

8. Very full; you ate a little too much, but it tasted really good.

9. Uncomfortable; you're too full. You're bloated and tired, and you don't feel great.

10. Stuffed; you're uncomfortable and maybe even nauseated. Never allow yourself to get to this point.

you reach level 5, but definitely no later than level 6. If you get to level 7, you've eaten too much. Anything above that is way too much and will sabotage your weight-loss efforts.

If you're not in the habit of eating regular meals and snacks, creating a food schedule that you use in conjunction with your journal can help you stay on track. Successful *Biggest Losers* learn over time that carefully planning their meals and snacks is one of the most important components of successful weight loss.

PLANNING REGULAR MEALS AND SNACKS

Trainer Jillian Michaels has a saying that has caught on among each season's contestants: "If you fail to plan, you plan to fail." Planning is crucial to just about every aspect of weight loss, from planning meals and snacks to planning exercise and adequate sleep. Part of planning includes making sure you have your journal with you at all times to record every meal and snack. Dan Evans of Season 5 advises, "Make sure you are totally conscious of what you're eating. Otherwise, it's easy for your inner fat person to sneak back out."

Breakfast

When it comes to breakfast, rule number one is: Eat it every day, no skipping. If you're not used to eating something within an hour of waking, you'll have to teach your body to reset its hunger signals. Try starting small and eating something simple, such as a bowl of fruit or a slice of whole grain toast with some almond butter. Try to include fiber and protein in your breakfast, which will keep you feeling full all morning.

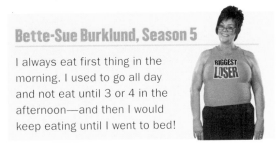

Bette-Sue Burklund, Season 5

I always eat first thing in the morning. I used to go all day and not eat until 3 or 4 in the afternoon—and then I would keep eating until I went to bed!

Lunch

It's easy to eat fast food in the car, buy lunch from a vending machine, or grab a handful of something from the fridge, but you'll probably make better food choices—and enjoy your meal more—if you do a little prep work ahead of time and use lunch as an opportunity to recharge for the second half of your day. As trainer Jillian Michaels points out, fueling your body with healthy food in the middle of the day will keep your metabolism on an even keel.

Make sure your lunch includes a combination of lean protein, complex carbs, and healthy fats. You might have a salad with lots of vegetables and a serving of lean protein, or a sandwich made with whole grain bread. You have a lot to accomplish in your afternoon, so feed yourself wisely!

Snacks

Snacks should be eaten midmorning and midafternoon, a few hours after you've had breakfast or lunch, when you're beginning to feel your energy wane. Try to eat something about every 3 to 4 hours, which will help keep cravings at bay, blood sugar stable, and energy up. Aim for a snack that combines one serving of carbohydrates (such as a piece of whole fruit) with a half

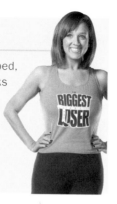

Amy Cremen, Season 6

Every night before you go to bed, prepare your lunch and snacks for the next day. Use snack-size zip-top bags for the correct portion sizes so you don't eat too much. This will help you avoid the drive-thru and the vending machine.

serving of protein (such as a low-fat cheese stick). Protein will help you feel full and satisfied, and a snack that combines protein with carbs will help keep your blood sugar stable.

When you're away from home, be sure to plan and pack your snacks for the day. Many *Biggest Losers* also find it helpful to keep preportioned snacks in the fridge in plastic bags or reusable containers—they're handy for preworkout pick-me-ups and postgym refueling.

Dinner

Take the time to slow down and enjoy your dinner. Plan your weekly menu based on your calorie budget and weight-loss goals. Write your shopping list on the weekend and make a supermarket run to ensure that you have everything you need for the week to come. Try to cook a few healthy meals on the weekend that you can refrigerate or freeze in individual portions and heat up as needed for a quick weeknight meal.

Dinner doesn't have to be a big, heavy meal. In fact, Season 5 winner Ali Vincent says she decides how light or substantial her dinner will be based on what she plans to do with the rest of her evening. Is she going to take a walk after dinner or go to a Pilates class? If so, she'll fuel

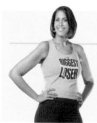

Heba Salama and Ed Brantley, Season 6

In your free time, prepare brown rice, quinoa, and whole wheat pasta—these items can be ready when you need them for a quick but balanced meal.

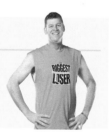

accordingly. Is she going to relax at home or catch up with friends? Then she'll eat lighter. Make modifications based on your lifestyle and calorie budget.

Liquid Calories

Your beverage of choice should always be water. If you're not already doing so, make sure to drink eight 8-ounce glasses of water a day to stay properly hydrated. This is especially important when you're changing your food habits and incorporating more fiber into your diet. Record your water intake in your journal each day to be sure you've met your quota.

Staying hydrated improves all bodily functions at the cellular level and helps your heart and kidneys work more efficiently. In addition, water carries glucose, nutrients, and dietary antioxidants to your tissues, resulting in an energy boost and other health benefits. And water actually helps regulate body temperature (especially important for people with poor circulation) and helps you feel full. In fact, some studies have shown that drinking a large glass of water 30 minutes before a meal can reduce calorie intake during the meal.

Neill Harmer, Season 5

Calories are like your daily allowance. If you have a coffee drink with whipped cream and chocolate (400 calories), you just spent a *big* part of your allowance on something that really wasn't needed. Spend your calories wisely.

In addition to water, you can have coffee, tea, low-fat or skim milk, and protein shakes on *The Biggest Loser* plan. Try to limit caffeine consumption to a minimum, however, and if you're drinking coffee or tea, it should never include syrup, whipped cream, or chocolate! On page 245 of the Appendix, you will find a chart that lists the caffeine content of common beverages. Don't forget to record *all* beverages you consume in your journal.

GET MOVING

As you know by now, weight loss is all about calories in and calories out. Calculating a calorie budget, planning your meals and snacks, and tracking what you eat are all great ways to make sure you're taking in the right number and right kind of calories. But what about that "calories out" part of the equation?

The contestants at the Ranch put in long, hard workouts every day. But you don't have to work out for hours with Bob and Jillian to see results. If you're not already active, start incorporating more activity into your day. Walk or bike instead of driving; take the stairs instead of the elevator; treat your dog to an extra-long walk. It doesn't matter how small you start—you just have to get moving.

If you already exercise moderately, consider increasing the duration (amount of time) and intensity (level of effort) of your workouts to see more results. If you typically walk or run on a treadmill for 30 minutes, try adding an incline, holding some hand weights, or increasing your time by 10 minutes. If you take a beginner yoga class once a week, ask yourself if you're ready to move to the intermediate level, or take the class twice week. The more you put into your fitness regimen, the more you'll get out of it.

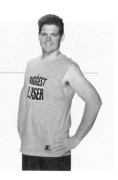

Daris George, Season 9 Finalist

Get into a routine and know what you have to do each day. Get up and get moving. It doesn't have to be at the gym—just take a walk!

Here are some tools to help you get moving, no matter what your fitness level is today.

Make a Plan

Studies show that people who plan ahead for their workouts are generally more successful than those who wing it. Decide when you want to work out and put it in your day planner. Earmark that time as yours. After you've exercised, record your accomplishments in this journal.

■ Set an alarm as a reminder to work out. Or schedule a reminder on your computer if that's where you spend most of your day.

■ Pack your gym bag the night before so that you can grab it and go in the morning.

Build a Team

At the Ranch, contestants are divided into teams to provide support and guidance for one another. You'll need that encouragement, too!

- Plan walking activities with your kids or encourage a friend to become an exercise buddy.
- Look for workout partners online through sites like BiggestLoserClub.com or through your local colleges, churches, and community centers.

Be Consistent

Experts suggest that it takes 21 days of consistent behavior to form a habit—so don't get discouraged after only a couple of days. Find small ways to stay active, and before you know it, your body will start to crave exercise.

Get FITTE

FITTE is a quick, handy acronym to help you remember all the elements of an exercise routine you need in order to improve your fitness. It's a good way, especially for beginners, to start thinking about working out. As you begin to make exercise a part of your lifestyle, you'll want to vary or increase some or all elements of the FITTE principle.

Frequency: How often you work out

Intensity: How hard you work out (measuring with a heart rate monitor or using rate of perceived exertion)

Time: The duration of your workout

Type: The kind of exercise you're doing

Enjoyment: How much pleasure you get out of the activity

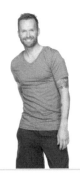

Biggest Loser Trainer Tip: Bob Harper

Incorporate weight training into your workout routine. You'll burn 8 to 10 calories a minute and boost your metabolism for an hour after your workout.

Frequency

The American Council on Exercise recommends 20 to 30 minutes of cardiovascular exercise 3 to 5 days a week (depending on intensity; a shorter workout duration calls for more intensity) and strength training at least twice a week. You can combine cardio and strength on some days or keep them separate.

Intensity: Load, Speed, and Effort

There are many ways to increase or decrease intensity.

- Load: This the amount of resistance you use in your workout. For strength training, you can use your own body weight as resistance or increase the load (and intensity) by adding weights.

- Speed: During your cardio workouts, you can amp up intensity by simply going faster. It will help you burn more calories and strengthen your heart. You can vary speed in strength exercises, too. When exercising with dumbbells, keep your speed under control to ensure that you never swing the weights.

- Effort: Adjusting this is one of the most common ways to vary intensity. How hard are you working? There are two ways to measure intensity. The most com-

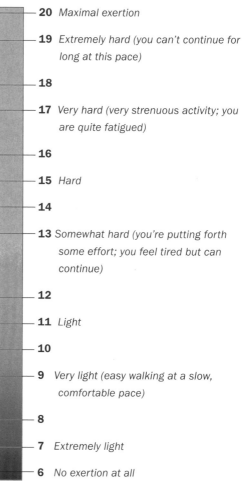

RATE OF PERCEIVED EXERTION SCALE

20 *Maximal exertion*

19 *Extremely hard (you can't continue for long at this pace)*

18

17 *Very hard (very strenuous activity; you are quite fatigued)*

16

15 *Hard*

14

13 *Somewhat hard (you're putting forth some effort; you feel tired but can continue)*

12

11 *Light*

10

9 *Very light (easy walking at a slow, comfortable pace)*

8

7 *Extremely light*

6 *No exertion at all*

mon is called rate of perceived exertion (RPE), and it is an easy-to-follow self-measurement. Use the rating scale on the opposite page to gauge how your body feels when you're working out. RPE ranges from 6 (no exertion at all) to 20 (maximal exertion).

Calculating Your Target Heart Rate

The rate of perceived exertion scale relates to your exercise heart rate as well. We all have a resting heart rate (our pulse rate when we're motionless), a maximum heart rate (the highest rate we should reach in a workout), and a target heart rate zone (for maximum fat burning). Your target heart rate—the rate that you should aim to achieve in your workouts—can be easily calculated, once you know your maximum heart rate. To find your maximum heart rate, follow this simple formula.

220 - your age = maximum heart rate

So, for a 35-year-old, the maximum heart rate is 185 (220 minus 35).

Now, to find your target heart rate zone, you're going to use the number you just calculated for your maximum heart rate.

Low end of target heart rate zone = maximum heart rate × 0.80

High end of target heart rate zone = maximum heart rate × 0.85

So, for the same 35-year-old . . .

■ The low end of the target heart rate zone (80 percent of maximum heart rate) would be 148 (185 × 0.80 = 148).

Biggest Loser Trainer Tip: Jillian Michaels

Always warm up for 5 minutes with light cardio, then do your resistance training. Follow your routine by stretching. Don't stretch before you're warmed up or you can risk injury.

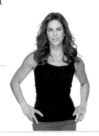

■ The high end of the target heart rate zone (85 percent of maximum heart rate) would be 157 (185 × 0.85 = 157).

This person should aim to keep his or her heart rate between 148 and 157 when exercising.

Studies have shown a correlation between rate of perceived exertion and heart rate, with heart rate equaling about 10 times the RPE you've reached. For example, if you're working out at an 11 on the RPE scale, your heart rate should be approximately 110. For a 35-year-old, for example, this would not be in the target heart rate zone. He or she would need to increase the intensity and be more in the 14-to-16 range to achieve the 148-to-157 target heart rate zone. Looking at the RPE scale, this makes sense, as that range represents "somewhat hard" to "hard."

Time

Time (or duration) is how long you actually exercise. We're all challenged to find time to exercise, but it's important to stick to your exercise schedule and put in as many minutes or hours as you can dedicate if you want to achieve your weight-loss goals.

Type

The type of exercise you choose will have a great impact on whether you can maintain a fitness program. If you prefer to fulfill your 30 minutes of aerobic exercise with cycling rather than walking, go ahead. Studies show that you'll be more likely to stick to an exercise program if you like what you're doing. Other options are swimming, jumping rope, and taking aerobics classes.

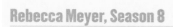

Rebecca Meyer, Season 8

Instead of hitting the refrigerator when you're upset, hit a boxing bag! All those endorphins really help, and you will feel so much better.

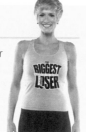

If you don't enjoy lifting dumbbells, try using tubing, elastic bands, medicine balls, weighted water balls, or a stability ball. (Go to BiggestLoser.com for products.)

Enjoyment

Season 4 finalist Julie Hadden has found a great, free way to exercise: She takes her kids to the park and climbs, slides, and plays! Inline skating, kickboxing, cycling, skiing, and surfing are all excellent activities that will keep you active and healthy. Take advantage of any class you can find that will introduce you to new ways to move your body.

USING YOUR FOOD JOURNAL

Using your food journal to track your calorie budget and record your progress will help you see your eating patterns more clearly, making it easy to discern which foods are helping you reach your goals and which foods trigger out-of-control eating or gains on the scale. As

Mike Morelli, Season 7 Finalist

Not everyone has the opportunity to be on *The Biggest Loser*. But everyone has the ability to change.

you learn which foods work best for you, make sure those foods are around when you need them. Keep them stocked in your pantry at home and, whenever possible, bring them with you on the go. Similarly, try to keep trigger foods out of your environment.

Each blank journal page is divided into two sections. In "What I Ate," you'll record your meals and snacks (and any accompanying beverages), noting the calorie count and the amount of carbohydrate, protein, and fat in each food. In "What I Did," you'll note the type and duration of any exercise that you do each day.

At the top of the page, you'll find a space to write your calorie goal for the day (based on your calorie budget calculation). Farther down, you'll also find a space to tally up the calories you consume each day and compare it with your goal calories, to see if you ate more or less than your budget allows.

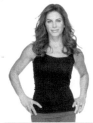

Biggest Loser Trainer Tip: Jillian Michaels

As you start stocking up your kitchen, do a junk-food sweep. Get rid of anything that might trigger an overeating episode. If the junk food's not around, you won't eat it.

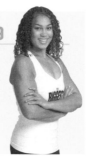

SunShine Hampton, Season 9

Working hard is a daily commitment. Each day, you have to get up and dedicate yourself to healthy eating and working out. There's no easy way, but there's the right way. And this is it.

The most important thing about keeping a food journal is getting into the habit of writing down everything you eat and drink, so that you get a better sense of what you're consuming each day and how many calories you're taking in. While it's also important to track your fat, carbohydrate, and protein intake, if doing so feels a little too overwhelming at first, it's ok to ease into things. Start by noting the calories in your meals and snacks, and once you get used to keeping the journal, you can become more meticulous about your tracking.

Each season at *The Biggest Loser* Ranch, the contestants are asked to write down their mantras. As the season progresses and things get tough, they turn to these words for inspiration and strength. A mantra can be as simple as a few words or as long as a few sentences; it might be a favorite quote, a personal motto, or a clearly articulated statement of purpose. Whatever form it takes, these mantras serve as sources of motivation and inspiration for *The Biggest Losers* when the going gets tough. On the opposite page, write down your mantra. You can also write it in a place where you're likely to see it every day—such as a note tucked into your wallet, posted on the fridge, or tacked to your office bulletin board. Keep your mantra in mind each day. It will remind you why you started on this journey—and why it's important to keep going.

MY MANTRA IS . . .

_____

_____

_____

_____

DATE:

CALORIE GOAL:

WHAT I ATE:

		Calories	Carbohydrate (45%)	Protein (30%)	Fat (25%)
BREAKFAST					
LUNCH					
DINNER					
SNACK 1					
SNACK 2					

TOTAL CALORIES: +/- GOAL CALORIES:

GLASSES OF WATER   ○ ○ ○ ○ ○ ○ ○ ○

WHAT I DID:

		Duration
EXERCISE		

DATE: _____

CALORIE GOAL: _____

WHAT I ATE:

	Calories	Carbohydrate (45%)	Protein (30%)	Fat (25%)
BREAKFAST				
LUNCH				
DINNER				
SNACK 1				
SNACK 2				

TOTAL CALORIES: _____ **+/- GOAL CALORIES:** _____

GLASSES OF WATER ○ ○ ○ ○ ○ ○ ○ ○

WHAT I DID:

	Duration
EXERCISE	

DATE: _____

CALORIE GOAL: _____

WHAT I ATE:

	Calories	Carbohydrate (45%)	Protein (30%)	Fat (25%)
BREAKFAST				
LUNCH				
DINNER				
SNACK 1				
SNACK 2				

TOTAL CALORIES: _____ **+/- GOAL CALORIES:** _____

GLASSES OF WATER ○ ○ ○ ○ ○ ○ ○ ○

WHAT I DID:

	Duration
EXERCISE	

DATE:

CALORIE GOAL:

WHAT I ATE:

		Calories	Carbohydrate (45%)	Protein (30%)	Fat (25%)
BREAKFAST					
LUNCH					
DINNER					
SNACK 1					
SNACK 2					

TOTAL CALORIES:	+/- GOAL CALORIES:

GLASSES OF WATER ○ ○ ○ ○ ○ ○ ○ ○

WHAT I DID:

		Duration
EXERCISE		

DATE: CALORIE GOAL:

WHAT I ATE:

		Calories	Carbohydrate (45%)	Protein (30%)	Fat (25%)
BREAKFAST					
LUNCH					
DINNER					
SNACK 1					
SNACK 2					

TOTAL CALORIES:	+/- GOAL CALORIES:

GLASSES OF WATER ○ ○ ○ ○ ○ ○ ○ ○

WHAT I DID:

		Duration
EXERCISE		

SOUTHERN START

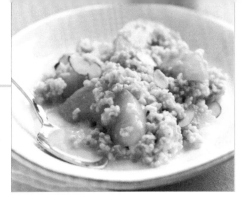

Season 8's Shay Sorrells says, "I just love cereal with sliced peaches and sliced almonds. Frozen fruit makes it possible to enjoy this combo year-round!" Its "peaches and cream" taste will satisfy anyone with a morning sweet tooth.

1	cup cooked steel-cut oats
¼	cup sliced frozen peaches
1	tablespoon slivered almonds
1	teaspoon vanilla extract
¼	cup Almond Breeze unsweetened vanilla almond milk
1	packet Truvia or other natural sweetener

Combine the oats, peaches, almonds, vanilla extract, almond milk, and sweetener in a cereal bowl and stir well. Microwave for 1 to 2 minutes.

Makes 1 serving

Per serving: 230 calories, 8 g protein, 34 g carbohydrates, 7 g fat (less than 1 g saturated), 0 mg cholesterol, 5 g fiber, 45 mg sodium

Recipe excerpted from *The Biggest Loser: 6 Weeks to a Healthier You*

For more ways to live *The Biggest Loser* lifestyle, go to biggestloser.com.

DATE: _____

CALORIE GOAL: _____

WHAT I ATE:

	Calories	Carbohydrate (45%)	Protein (30%)	Fat (25%)
BREAKFAST				
LUNCH				
DINNER				
SNACK 1				
SNACK 2				

TOTAL CALORIES: _____ **+/- GOAL CALORIES:** _____

GLASSES OF WATER ◯ ◯ ◯ ◯ ◯ ◯ ◯ ◯

WHAT I DID:

	Duration
EXERCISE	

DATE:

CALORIE GOAL:

WHAT I ATE:

		Calories	Carbohydrate (45%)	Protein (30%)	Fat (25%)
BREAKFAST					
LUNCH					
DINNER					
SNACK 1					
SNACK 2					

TOTAL CALORIES:	+/- GOAL CALORIES:

GLASSES OF WATER ○ ○ ○ ○ ○ ○ ○ ○

WHAT I DID:

		Duration
EXERCISE		

DATE: _____

CALORIE GOAL: _____

WHAT I ATE:

		Calories	Carbohydrate (45%)	Protein (30%)	Fat (25%)
BREAKFAST					
LUNCH					
DINNER					
SNACK 1					
SNACK 2					

TOTAL CALORIES: _____ **+/- GOAL CALORIES:** _____

GLASSES OF WATER ○ ○ ○ ○ ○ ○ ○ ○

WHAT I DID:

		Duration
EXERCISE		

DATE:

CALORIE GOAL:

WHAT I ATE:

	Calories	Carbohydrate (45%)	Protein (30%)	Fat (25%)
BREAKFAST				
LUNCH				
DINNER				
SNACK 1				
SNACK 2				

TOTAL CALORIES: **+/- GOAL CALORIES:**

GLASSES OF WATER   ○ ○ ○ ○ ○ ○ ○ ○

WHAT I DID:

	Duration
EXERCISE	

DATE:

CALORIE GOAL:

WHAT I ATE:

	Calories	Carbohydrate (45%)	Protein (30%)	Fat (25%)
BREAKFAST				
LUNCH				
DINNER				
SNACK 1				
SNACK 2				

TOTAL CALORIES: **+/- GOAL CALORIES:**

GLASSES OF WATER ○ ○ ○ ○ ○ ○ ○ ○

WHAT I DID:

	Duration
EXERCISE	

EGG WHITE BITES

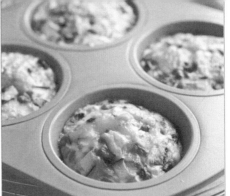

Season 3's Jen Eisenbarth and her family enjoy the versatility of this recipe as well as the ease of preparation. Get creative and invent your own favorite bites!

2	cups grated or finely chopped vegetables (asparagus, bell peppers, carrots, mushrooms, onion, spinach, yellow squash, zucchini)
18	egg whites, or 2¼ cups egg whites or egg substitute
	Salt-free seasoning to taste
	Ground black pepper to taste
¼	cup grated low-fat Cheddar, Jack, or mozzarella cheese

Position a rack in the center of the oven and preheat the oven to 350°F. Lightly coat two 6-cup muffin pans with olive oil cooking spray.

Spray a nonstick skillet with cooking spray and cook the vegetables briefly, until they reach the desired crispness or tenderness.

Place a small nest of vegetables in the bottom of each muffin cup, then fill the cups ¾ full with egg whites. Add salt-free seasoning, black pepper, and other seasoning as desired. Sprinkle a small amount of cheese over each cup.

Bake the eggs for about 10 minutes, until they are just set. Cool in the pans.

Makes 12 (1-bite) servings

Per serving: 40 calories, 6 g protein, 3 g carbohydrates, less than 1 g fat (0 g saturated), 10 mg cholesterol, 1 g fiber, 110 mg sodium

DATE:

CALORIE GOAL:

WHAT I ATE:

	Calories	Carbohydrate (45%)	Protein (30%)	Fat (25%)
BREAKFAST				
LUNCH				
DINNER				
SNACK 1				
SNACK 2				

TOTAL CALORIES: **+/- GOAL CALORIES:**

GLASSES OF WATER ◯ ◯ ◯ ◯ ◯ ◯ ◯ ◯

WHAT I DID:

	Duration
EXERCISE	

DATE:

WHAT I ATE:

	Calories	Carbohydrate (45%)	Protein (30%)	Fat (25%)
BREAKFAST				
LUNCH				
DINNER				
SNACK 1				
SNACK 2				

TOTAL CALORIES:	**+/- GOAL CALORIES:**
GLASSES OF WATER	○ ○ ○ ○ ○ ○ ○ ○

WHAT I DID:

	Duration
EXERCISE	

DATE:

CALORIE GOAL:

WHAT I ATE:

	Calories	Carbohydrate (45%)	Protein (30%)	Fat (25%)
BREAKFAST				
LUNCH				
DINNER				
SNACK 1				
SNACK 2				

TOTAL CALORIES: +/- GOAL CALORIES:

GLASSES OF WATER   ○ ○ ○ ○ ○ ○ ○ ○

WHAT I DID:

	Duration
EXERCISE	

DATE:

CALORIE GOAL:

WHAT I ATE:

	Calories	Carbohydrate (45%)	Protein (30%)	Fat (25%)
BREAKFAST				
LUNCH				
DINNER				
SNACK 1				
SNACK 2				

TOTAL CALORIES: +/- GOAL CALORIES:

GLASSES OF WATER ○ ○ ○ ○ ○ ○ ○ ○

WHAT I DID:

	Duration
EXERCISE	

DATE:

CALORIE GOAL:

WHAT I ATE:

		Calories	Carbohydrate (45%)	Protein (30%)	Fat (25%)
BREAKFAST					
LUNCH					
DINNER					
SNACK 1					
SNACK 2					

TOTAL CALORIES:	+/- GOAL CALORIES:
GLASSES OF WATER	○ ○ ○ ○ ○ ○ ○ ○

WHAT I DID:

	Duration
EXERCISE	

SUNRISE SHAKE

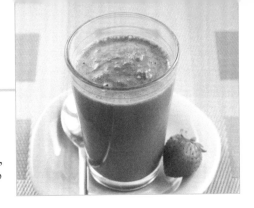

Like many other contestants, Season 9's Stephanie Anderson has a major sweet tooth. Though she likes to make this shake for breakfast, it's a great recovery drink after a workout, too, since it contains 7 grams of protein to help rebuild tired muscles.

1	cup Almond Breeze unsweetened vanilla almond milk
½	banana
½	cup sliced strawberries, frozen or fresh
2	scoops (4 tablespoons) *The Biggest Loser* chocolate protein powder
1	tablespoon unsweetened cocoa powder
1	teaspoon vanilla extract
1	package Truvia or other natural sweetener
1	cup ice

Combine the almond milk, banana, strawberries, protein powder, cocoa powder, vanilla extract, sweetener, and ice in a blender. Blend or puree until smooth. Pour into glasses and serve immediately.

Makes 2 (1½-cup) servings

Per serving: 100 calories, 7 g protein, 19 g carbohydrates, 2 g fat (0 g saturated), 0 mg cholesterol, 8 g fiber, 85 mg sodium

DATE:

CALORIE GOAL:

WHAT I ATE:

	Calories	Carbohydrate (45%)	Protein (30%)	Fat (25%)
BREAKFAST				
LUNCH				
DINNER				
SNACK 1				
SNACK 2				

TOTAL CALORIES: **+/- GOAL CALORIES:**

GLASSES OF WATER   ○ ○ ○ ○ ○ ○ ○ ○

WHAT I DID:

	Duration
EXERCISE	

DATE:

CALORIE GOAL:

WHAT I ATE:

		Calories	Carbohydrate (45%)	Protein (30%)	Fat (25%)
BREAKFAST					
LUNCH					
DINNER					
SNACK 1					
SNACK 2					

TOTAL CALORIES:	+/- GOAL CALORIES:
GLASSES OF WATER	○ ○ ○ ○ ○ ○ ○ ○

WHAT I DID:

		Duration
EXERCISE		

DATE:

CALORIE GOAL:

WHAT I ATE:

		Calories	Carbohydrate (45%)	Protein (30%)	Fat (25%)
BREAKFAST					
LUNCH					
DINNER					
SNACK 1					
SNACK 2					

TOTAL CALORIES: **+/- GOAL CALORIES:**

GLASSES OF WATER ○ ○ ○ ○ ○ ○ ○ ○

WHAT I DID:

	Duration
EXERCISE	

DATE:

CALORIE GOAL:

WHAT I ATE:

		Calories	Carbohydrate (45%)	Protein (30%)	Fat (25%)
BREAKFAST					
LUNCH					
DINNER					
SNACK 1					
SNACK 2					

TOTAL CALORIES:	+/- GOAL CALORIES:

GLASSES OF WATER	○ ○ ○ ○ ○ ○ ○ ○

WHAT I DID:

	Duration
EXERCISE	

DATE:

CALORIE GOAL:

WHAT I ATE:

		Calories	Carbohydrate (45%)	Protein (30%)	Fat (25%)
BREAKFAST					
LUNCH					
DINNER					
SNACK 1					
SNACK 2					

TOTAL CALORIES:	+/- GOAL CALORIES:

GLASSES OF WATER	○ ○ ○ ○ ○ ○ ○ ○

WHAT I DID:

		Duration
EXERCISE		

GOLDEN FLAXJACKS

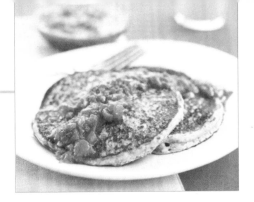

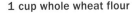

Whole grains add texture and flavor to any recipe, and flaxseed contains heart-healthy omega-3s. Cook your flaxjacks over moderate heat so they don't burn; the flaxseed makes them brown more quickly.

1 cup whole wheat flour

½ cup stone-ground cornmeal

2 tablespoons wheat bran or oat bran

2 tablespoons flaxseed meal (see note)

2 teaspoons baking powder

½ teaspoon salt

2 large egg whites

1¾ cups fat-free or 1% milk

2 tablespoons olive oil or canola oil

½ teaspoon vanilla extract

In a large mixing bowl, combine the flour, cornmeal, bran, flaxseed meal, baking powder, and salt. Set aside.

In a small mixing bowl or blender, whisk together the egg whites, milk, oil, and vanilla extract until smooth. Make a well in the center of the dry ingredients. Pour the liquid mixture into the well and stir until just combined. Allow the batter to stand for about 30 minutes or overnight in the refrigerator. Add more milk, if needed, to obtain batter the consistency of thick cream.

Heat a nonstick griddle or nonstick skillet (coated with cooking spray if necessary) to medium heat. For each flaxjack, pour a scant ¼ cup of batter onto the griddle. Cook until the flaxjacks are puffed and dry around the edges. Turn and cook the other side until golden brown.

Note: If you can't find flaxseed meal, you can grind whole flaxseeds yourself in a spice grinder or clean coffee grinder. Grind to the consistency of cornmeal. Four teaspoons of whole flaxseeds yields approximately 2 tablespoons of flaxseed meal.

Makes 8 servings of 2 (4") flaxjacks

Per serving: 160 calories, 6 g protein, 23 g carbohydrates, 5 g fat (1 g saturated), 0 mg cholesterol, 4 g fiber, 320 mg sodium

DATE:

CALORIE GOAL:

WHAT I ATE:

	Calories	Carbohydrate (45%)	Protein (30%)	Fat (25%)
BREAKFAST				
LUNCH				
DINNER				
SNACK 1				
SNACK 2				

TOTAL CALORIES: **+/- GOAL CALORIES:**

GLASSES OF WATER ○ ○ ○ ○ ○ ○ ○ ○

WHAT I DID:

	Duration
EXERCISE	

DATE: _____

CALORIE GOAL: _____

WHAT I ATE:

		Calories	Carbohydrate (45%)	Protein (30%)	Fat (25%)
BREAKFAST					
LUNCH					
DINNER					
SNACK 1					
SNACK 2					

TOTAL CALORIES: _____ **+/- GOAL CALORIES:** _____

GLASSES OF WATER ○ ○ ○ ○ ○ ○ ○ ○

WHAT I DID:

		Duration
EXERCISE		

DATE:

CALORIE GOAL:

WHAT I ATE:

	Calories	Carbohydrate (45%)	Protein (30%)	Fat (25%)
BREAKFAST				
LUNCH				
DINNER				
SNACK 1				
SNACK 2				

TOTAL CALORIES: **+/- GOAL CALORIES:**

GLASSES OF WATER ○ ○ ○ ○ ○ ○ ○ ○

WHAT I DID:

	Duration
EXERCISE	

DATE: _____

CALORIE GOAL: _____

WHAT I ATE:

		Calories	Carbohydrate (45%)	Protein (30%)	Fat (25%)
BREAKFAST					
LUNCH					
DINNER					
SNACK 1					
SNACK 2					

TOTAL CALORIES: _____ **+/- GOAL CALORIES:** _____

GLASSES OF WATER ○ ○ ○ ○ ○ ○ ○ ○

WHAT I DID:

		Duration
EXERCISE		

DATE:

CALORIE GOAL:

WHAT I ATE:

	Calories	Carbohydrate (45%)	Protein (30%)	Fat (25%)
BREAKFAST				
LUNCH				
DINNER				
SNACK 1				
SNACK 2				

TOTAL CALORIES: **+/- GOAL CALORIES:**

GLASSES OF WATER ○ ○ ○ ○ ○ ○ ○ ○

WHAT I DID:

	Duration
EXERCISE	

BERRY-LICIOUS OATMEAL

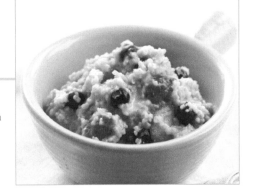

Season 8's Shay Sorrells says, "I'm really busy, so I always buy precooked steel-cut oats, which makes this an easy breakfast recipe." You can use any combination of fresh or frozen (and thawed) berries for this delicious, fruit-packed start to your day.

1	cup cooked steel-cut oats
2	tablespoons fresh or frozen blueberries
2	tablespoons fresh or frozen raspberries
½	cup sliced strawberries
1	teaspoon vanilla extract
¼	cup Almond Breeze unsweetened vanilla almond milk
1	packet Truvia or other natural sweetener

Combine the oats, berries, vanilla, almond milk, and sweetener in a cereal bowl and stir well. Microwave for 1 to 2 minutes and serve.

Makes 1 serving

Per serving: 220 calories, 7 g protein, 39 g carbohydrates (8 g sugars), 4 g fat (0 g saturated), 0 mg cholesterol, 7 g fiber, 50 mg sodium

DATE: _____

CALORIE GOAL: _____

WHAT I ATE:

		Calories	Carbohydrate (45%)	Protein (30%)	Fat (25%)
BREAKFAST					
LUNCH					
DINNER					
SNACK 1					
SNACK 2					

TOTAL CALORIES:	**+/- GOAL CALORIES:**

GLASSES OF WATER ○ ○ ○ ○ ○ ○ ○ ○

WHAT I DID:

		Duration
EXERCISE		

DATE:

CALORIE GOAL:

WHAT I ATE:

		Calories	Carbohydrate (45%)	Protein (30%)	Fat (25%)
BREAKFAST					
LUNCH					
DINNER					
SNACK 1					
SNACK 2					

TOTAL CALORIES: **+/- GOAL CALORIES:**

GLASSES OF WATER   ○ ○ ○ ○ ○ ○ ○ ○

WHAT I DID:

	Duration
EXERCISE	

DATE:

CALORIE GOAL:

WHAT I ATE:

		Calories	Carbohydrate (45%)	Protein (30%)	Fat (25%)
BREAKFAST					
LUNCH					
DINNER					
SNACK 1					
SNACK 2					

TOTAL CALORIES: **+/- GOAL CALORIES:**

GLASSES OF WATER   ○ ○ ○ ○ ○ ○ ○ ○

WHAT I DID:

	Duration
EXERCISE	

DATE:

WHAT I ATE:

	Calories	Carbohydrate (45%)	Protein (30%)	Fat (25%)
BREAKFAST				
LUNCH				
DINNER				
SNACK 1				
SNACK 2				

TOTAL CALORIES: **+/- GOAL CALORIES:**

GLASSES OF WATER   ○ ○ ○ ○ ○ ○ ○ ○

WHAT I DID:

	Duration
EXERCISE	

DATE: _____

CALORIE GOAL: _____

WHAT I ATE:

		Calories	Carbohydrate (45%)	Protein (30%)	Fat (25%)
BREAKFAST					
LUNCH					
DINNER					
SNACK 1					
SNACK 2					

TOTAL CALORIES: _____ **+/- GOAL CALORIES:** _____

GLASSES OF WATER ○ ○ ○ ○ ○ ○ ○ ○

WHAT I DID:

		Duration
EXERCISE		

HAM AND CHEESE BREAKFAST MELT

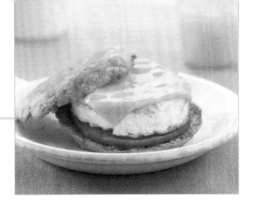

You can add mustard or a slice of tomato to customize this sandwich. It reheats well, too, so you might want to make two at a time and warm the second one the next day!

1	Thomas' Light Whole Grain English muffin, split
1	slice (1 ounce) lean, low-sodium ham or lean Canadian bacon
2	egg whites
1	slice low- or reduced-fat Cheddar cheese
	Salt and pepper to taste

Coat an egg ring (see note) with olive oil cooking spray.

Toast the muffin halves until they're lightly browned. While the muffin toasts, warm the ham for about 1 minute in a small nonstick skillet. Remove the ham from the skillet and place it on half of the toasted English muffin. Cover to keep it warm.

Place the prepared egg ring in the nonstick skillet over medium heat. Pour the egg whites into the ring. Cover the pan and cook over medium heat for about 3 minutes, or until the egg is nearly set. Run a knife or spatula around the inside edge of the ring to break the egg loose. Remove the ring. Flip the egg over and cook it for about 30 seconds longer, or until done.

Place the egg on top of the ham and season with salt and pepper. While the egg is piping hot, lay the cheese over it. Top with the remaining muffin half. Serve hot.

Note: If you don't have an egg ring, you can use the ring from a wide-mouthed canning jar.

Makes 1 serving

Per serving: 230 calories, 25 g protein, 25 g carbohydrates, 6 g fat (2 g saturated), 20 mg cholesterol, 8 g fiber, 570 mg sodium

DATE: _____

CALORIE GOAL: _____

WHAT I ATE:

	Calories	Carbohydrate (45%)	Protein (30%)	Fat (25%)
BREAKFAST				
LUNCH				
DINNER				
SNACK 1				
SNACK 2				

TOTAL CALORIES: _____ **+/- GOAL CALORIES:** _____

GLASSES OF WATER ○ ○ ○ ○ ○ ○ ○ ○

WHAT I DID:

	Duration
EXERCISE	

DATE:

CALORIE GOAL:

WHAT I ATE:

	Calories	Carbohydrate (45%)	Protein (30%)	Fat (25%)
BREAKFAST				
LUNCH				
DINNER				
SNACK 1				
SNACK 2				

TOTAL CALORIES: +/- GOAL CALORIES:

GLASSES OF WATER ○ ○ ○ ○ ○ ○ ○ ○

WHAT I DID:

	Duration
EXERCISE	

DATE:

CALORIE GOAL:

WHAT I ATE:

	Calories	Carbohydrate (45%)	Protein (30%)	Fat (25%)
BREAKFAST				
LUNCH				
DINNER				
SNACK 1				
SNACK 2				

TOTAL CALORIES: **+/- GOAL CALORIES:**

GLASSES OF WATER ○ ○ ○ ○ ○ ○ ○ ○

WHAT I DID:

	Duration
EXERCISE	

DATE: _____

CALORIE GOAL: _____

WHAT I ATE:

	Calories	Carbohydrate (45%)	Protein (30%)	Fat (25%)
BREAKFAST				
LUNCH				
DINNER				
SNACK 1				
SNACK 2				

TOTAL CALORIES: _____ **+/- GOAL CALORIES:** _____

GLASSES OF WATER ○ ○ ○ ○ ○ ○ ○ ○

WHAT I DID:

	Duration
EXERCISE	

DATE: _____

CALORIE GOAL:

WHAT I ATE:

	Calories	Carbohydrate (45%)	Protein (30%)	Fat (25%)
BREAKFAST				
LUNCH				
DINNER				
SNACK 1				
SNACK 2				

TOTAL CALORIES: _____ **+/- GOAL CALORIES:** _____

GLASSES OF WATER ○ ○ ○ ○ ○ ○ ○ ○

WHAT I DID:

	Duration
EXERCISE	

SPICY ALMOND CHAI

The fragrance of masala chai is as intoxicating as its complex flavor. Chai is traditionally prepared by steeping spices in hot water and milk before adding black tea, but this rendition uses unsweetened almond milk and green tea instead. Delicious hot or cold, it takes just minutes to prepare.

4	cups water
6	(¼"-thick) slices peeled fresh ginger
½	teaspoon ground cardamom
1	(3") cinnamon stick
6	whole cloves
6	green tea bags
2	cups unsweetened almond milk

In a small saucepan over medium heat, combine the water, ginger, cardamom, cinnamon, and cloves. Bring to a boil, then reduce the heat and simmer for about 3 minutes. Remove from the heat. Steep the tea bags in the spice mixture for 5 minutes. Strain the mixture into a container and store for up to 1 week in the refrigerator.

To serve, combine the tea concentrate with the almond milk in a small saucepan. Simmer over low heat, but do not boil. Sweeten if desired. (To prepare a single cup, mix ⅔ cup hot tea concentrate with ⅓ cup hot almond milk.)

Makes 6 (1-cup) servings

Per serving: 15 calories, 0 g protein, 1 g carbohydrates, 1 g fat (0 g saturated), 0 mg cholesterol, 0 g fiber, 60 mg sodium

DATE:

CALORIE GOAL:

WHAT I ATE:

	Calories	Carbohydrate (45%)	Protein (30%)	Fat (25%)
BREAKFAST				
LUNCH				
DINNER				
SNACK 1				
SNACK 2				

TOTAL CALORIES: 　　　　+/- GOAL CALORIES:

GLASSES OF WATER　○ ○ ○ ○ ○ ○ ○ ○

WHAT I DID:

	Duration
EXERCISE	

DATE:

CALORIE GOAL:

WHAT I ATE:

	Calories	Carbohydrate (45%)	Protein (30%)	Fat (25%)
BREAKFAST				
LUNCH				
DINNER				
SNACK 1				
SNACK 2				

TOTAL CALORIES: **+/- GOAL CALORIES:**

GLASSES OF WATER   ○ ○ ○ ○ ○ ○ ○ ○

WHAT I DID:

		Duration
EXERCISE		

DATE:

CALORIE GOAL:

WHAT I ATE:

	Calories	Carbohydrate (45%)	Protein (30%)	Fat (25%)
BREAKFAST				
LUNCH				
DINNER				
SNACK 1				
SNACK 2				

TOTAL CALORIES: **+/- GOAL CALORIES:**

GLASSES OF WATER ○ ○ ○ ○ ○ ○ ○ ○

WHAT I DID:

	Duration
EXERCISE	

DATE: _____

CALORIE GOAL: _____

WHAT I ATE:

		Calories	Carbohydrate (45%)	Protein (30%)	Fat (25%)
BREAKFAST					
LUNCH					
DINNER					
SNACK 1					
SNACK 2					

TOTAL CALORIES: _____   **+/- GOAL CALORIES:** _____

GLASSES OF WATER ◯ ◯ ◯ ◯ ◯ ◯ ◯ ◯

WHAT I DID:

	Duration
EXERCISE	

DATE: _____

CALORIE GOAL: _____

WHAT I ATE:

		Calories	Carbohydrate (45%)	Protein (30%)	Fat (25%)
BREAKFAST					
LUNCH					
DINNER					
SNACK 1					
SNACK 2					

TOTAL CALORIES: _____ **+/- GOAL CALORIES:** _____

GLASSES OF WATER ○ ○ ○ ○ ○ ○ ○ ○

WHAT I DID:

	Duration
EXERCISE	

MIXED BERRY SMOOTHIE

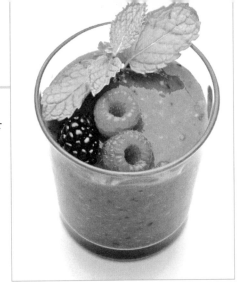

This refreshing smoothie is served to guests at *The Biggest Loser* Resort at Fitness Ridge. After a tough workout, resort guests cool down by sipping on this spa-quality pick-me-up that provides protein and potassium to help repair muscle and restore electrolytes. Whip up this simple smoothie in your blender and you'll feel like you're at the resort, too!

1	cup frozen blueberries
1	cup frozen strawberries
1	cup frozen raspberries
½	cup soy milk
1	banana
½	cup tofu mori nu light silken
1	teaspoon cinnamon
1	teaspoon vanilla extract

Combine the frozen berries, milk, banana, tofu, cinnamon, and vanilla extract in a blender. Blend or puree until smooth. Pour into glasses and serve immediately.

Makes 4 servings

Per serving: 195 calories, 4 g protein, 49 g carbohydrates, 3 g fat (0 g saturated), 0 mg cholesterol, 4 g fiber, 61 mg sodium

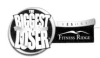

For more ways to live *The Biggest Loser* lifestyle, go to biggestloser.com.

DATE: _____

CALORIE GOAL: _____

WHAT I ATE:

	Calories	Carbohydrate (45%)	Protein (30%)	Fat (25%)
BREAKFAST				
LUNCH				
DINNER				
SNACK 1				
SNACK 2				

TOTAL CALORIES:	+/- GOAL CALORIES:
GLASSES OF WATER	○ ○ ○ ○ ○ ○ ○ ○

WHAT I DID:

	Duration
EXERCISE	

DATE:

CALORIE GOAL:

WHAT I ATE:

	Calories	Carbohydrate (45%)	Protein (30%)	Fat (25%)
BREAKFAST				
LUNCH				
DINNER				
SNACK 1				
SNACK 2				

TOTAL CALORIES:	+/- GOAL CALORIES:
GLASSES OF WATER	○ ○ ○ ○ ○ ○ ○ ○

WHAT I DID:

	Duration
EXERCISE	

DATE: _____

CALORIE GOAL: _____

WHAT I ATE:

	Calories	Carbohydrate (45%)	Protein (30%)	Fat (25%)
BREAKFAST				
LUNCH				
DINNER				
SNACK 1				
SNACK 2				

TOTAL CALORIES: _____ **+/- GOAL CALORIES:** _____

GLASSES OF WATER ○ ○ ○ ○ ○ ○ ○ ○

WHAT I DID:

	Duration
EXERCISE	

DATE:

CALORIE GOAL:

WHAT I ATE:

	Calories	Carbohydrate (45%)	Protein (30%)	Fat (25%)
BREAKFAST				
LUNCH				
DINNER				
SNACK 1				
SNACK 2				

TOTAL CALORIES: **+/- GOAL CALORIES:**

GLASSES OF WATER ○ ○ ○ ○ ○ ○ ○ ○

WHAT I DID:

	Duration
EXERCISE	

DATE:

CALORIE GOAL:

WHAT I ATE:

	Calories	Carbohydrate (45%)	Protein (30%)	Fat (25%)
BREAKFAST				
LUNCH				
DINNER				
SNACK 1				
SNACK 2				

TOTAL CALORIES:	+/- GOAL CALORIES:
GLASSES OF WATER	○ ○ ○ ○ ○ ○ ○ ○

WHAT I DID:

	Duration
EXERCISE	

TRAIL CORN

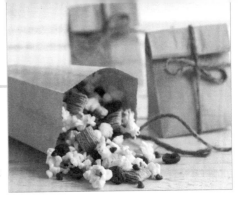

While traditional prepackaged trail mix usually contains healthy ingredients, it also tends to have a lot of fat. This version has much less fat and a bit more fiber. If you're not eating the trail corn immediately, it will stay freshest if you store the bags in a resealable plastic container.

4	**cups air-popped popcorn**
½	**cup high-fiber, low-sugar cereal squares (such as Quaker Oatmeal Squares)**
½	**cup dried red fruit (such as dried cherries or dried cranberries)**
2	**tablespoons mini chocolate chips**

In assembly line fashion, place 1 cup popcorn into each of 4 sandwich-size resealable plastic bags, followed by 2 tablespoons cereal, 2 tablespoons dried fruit, and ½ tablespoon chocolate chips. Seal each bag and shake it to distribute the ingredients evenly. The bags can be stored in an airtight container for up to 3 days.

Makes 4 (about 1¼-cup) servings

Per serving: 152 calories, 3 g protein, 29 g carbohydrates, 3 g fat (1 g saturated), 0 mg cholesterol, 4 g fiber, 37 mg sodium

DATE: | CALORIE GOAL:

WHAT I ATE:

		Calories	Carbohydrate (45%)	Protein (30%)	Fat (25%)
BREAKFAST					
LUNCH					
DINNER					
SNACK 1					
SNACK 2					

TOTAL CALORIES:	+/- GOAL CALORIES:
GLASSES OF WATER	○ ○ ○ ○ ○ ○ ○ ○

WHAT I DID:

EXERCISE	Duration

DATE: _____

CALORIE GOAL: _____

WHAT I ATE:

	Calories	Carbohydrate (45%)	Protein (30%)	Fat (25%)
BREAKFAST				
LUNCH				
DINNER				
SNACK 1				
SNACK 2				

TOTAL CALORIES: _____   **+/- GOAL CALORIES:** _____

GLASSES OF WATER   ○ ○ ○ ○ ○ ○ ○ ○

WHAT I DID:

	Duration
EXERCISE	

DATE:

CALORIE GOAL:

WHAT I ATE:

	Calories	Carbohydrate (45%)	Protein (30%)	Fat (25%)
BREAKFAST				
LUNCH				
DINNER				
SNACK 1				
SNACK 2				

TOTAL CALORIES: +/- GOAL CALORIES:

GLASSES OF WATER ○ ○ ○ ○ ○ ○ ○ ○

WHAT I DID:

	Duration
EXERCISE	

DATE:

CALORIE GOAL:

WHAT I ATE:

	Calories	Carbohydrate (45%)	Protein (30%)	Fat (25%)
BREAKFAST				
LUNCH				
DINNER				
SNACK 1				
SNACK 2				

TOTAL CALORIES: +/- GOAL CALORIES:

GLASSES OF WATER   ○ ○ ○ ○ ○ ○ ○ ○

WHAT I DID:

	Duration
EXERCISE	

DATE:

CALORIE GOAL:

WHAT I ATE:

	Calories	Carbohydrate (45%)	Protein (30%)	Fat (25%)
BREAKFAST				
LUNCH				
DINNER				
SNACK 1				
SNACK 2				

TOTAL CALORIES: **+/- GOAL CALORIES:**

GLASSES OF WATER ○ ○ ○ ○ ○ ○ ○ ○

WHAT I DID:

	Duration
EXERCISE	

EDAMAMMUS

This dip, which is like a hummus but made with edamame instead of chickpeas, is very versatile. You can serve it with your favorite veggies, such as carrots or celery, and it's also great with toasted whole wheat pita triangles or your favorite high-fiber whole wheat crackers.

8	ounces (about 1½ cups) cooked shelled edamame, cooled
2½	tablespoons lemon juice
2	medium cloves garlic, coarsely chopped
1	tablespoon fresh flat-leaf parsley, coarsely chopped
¼	teaspoon salt
1	teaspoon extra-virgin olive oil
3	tablespoons fat-free plain yogurt

In the bowl of a food processor fitted with a chopping blade, combine the edamame, lemon juice, garlic, parsley, and salt. Process until the mixture is pastelike and the edamame is finely chopped, scraping down the sides of the bowl as necessary. With the food processor on, slowly drizzle the oil through the top until well mixed. Add the yogurt and process until just combined. Serve immediately or refrigerate in an airtight container for up to 3 days.

Makes 5 (about ¼-cup) servings

Per serving: 66 calories, 5 g protein, 6 g carbohydrates, 3 g fat (trace saturated), trace cholesterol, 2 g fiber, 125 mg sodium

DATE: _____

CALORIE GOAL: _____

WHAT I ATE:

	Calories	Carbohydrate (45%)	Protein (30%)	Fat (25%)
BREAKFAST				
LUNCH				
DINNER				
SNACK 1				
SNACK 2				

TOTAL CALORIES: _____ **+/- GOAL CALORIES:** _____

GLASSES OF WATER ○ ○ ○ ○ ○ ○ ○ ○

WHAT I DID:

	Duration
EXERCISE	

DATE:

CALORIE GOAL:

WHAT I ATE:

	Calories	Carbohydrate (45%)	Protein (30%)	Fat (25%)
BREAKFAST				
LUNCH				
DINNER				
SNACK 1				
SNACK 2				

TOTAL CALORIES: **+/- GOAL CALORIES:**

GLASSES OF WATER ○ ○ ○ ○ ○ ○ ○ ○

WHAT I DID:

	Duration
EXERCISE	

DATE:

CALORIE GOAL:

WHAT I ATE:

		Calories	Carbohydrate (45%)	Protein (30%)	Fat (25%)
BREAKFAST					
LUNCH					
DINNER					
SNACK 1					
SNACK 2					

TOTAL CALORIES: **+/- GOAL CALORIES:**

GLASSES OF WATER ○ ○ ○ ○ ○ ○ ○ ○

WHAT I DID:

		Duration
EXERCISE		

DATE:

CALORIE GOAL:

WHAT I ATE:

	Calories	Carbohydrate (45%)	Protein (30%)	Fat (25%)
BREAKFAST				
LUNCH				
DINNER				
SNACK 1				
SNACK 2				

TOTAL CALORIES: **+/- GOAL CALORIES:**

GLASSES OF WATER   ◯ ◯ ◯ ◯ ◯ ◯ ◯ ◯

WHAT I DID:

		Duration
EXERCISE		

DATE:

CALORIE GOAL:

WHAT I ATE:

	Calories	Carbohydrate (45%)	Protein (30%)	Fat (25%)
BREAKFAST				
LUNCH				
DINNER				
SNACK 1				
SNACK 2				

TOTAL CALORIES: **+/- GOAL CALORIES:**

GLASSES OF WATER ○ ○ ○ ○ ○ ○ ○ ○

WHAT I DID:

	Duration
EXERCISE	

FROSTY ORANGE PROTEIN BLAST

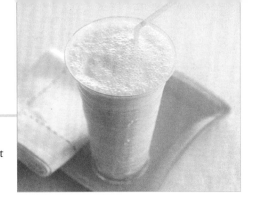

This creamy protein drink uses frozen orange juice concentrate to intensify the flavor without relying on additional sweeteners. It's a great postworkout snack.

2	cups unsweetened vanilla almond milk
1	(6-ounce) can frozen orange juice concentrate
1	cup fat-free Greek-style plain yogurt
1	teaspoon vanilla extract
2	scoops (4 tablespoons) *The Biggest Loser* vanilla protein powder
16	ice cubes

Add the almond milk, juice concentrate, yogurt, vanilla extract, protein powder, and ice to a blender. Blend until smooth.

Leftovers can be poured into small resealable plastic bags and stored in the freezer. Thaw slightly and blend before serving.

Makes 4 (1¼-cup) servings

Per serving: 140 calories, 10 g protein, 23 g carbohydrates, 2 g fat (0 g saturated), 0 mg cholesterol, 4 g fiber, 135 mg sodium

DATE: _____

CALORIE GOAL: _____

WHAT I ATE:

		Calories	Carbohydrate (45%)	Protein (30%)	Fat (25%)
BREAKFAST					
LUNCH					
DINNER					
SNACK 1					
SNACK 2					

TOTAL CALORIES: _____ **+/- GOAL CALORIES:** _____

GLASSES OF WATER ○ ○ ○ ○ ○ ○ ○ ○

WHAT I DID:

		Duration
EXERCISE		

DATE:

CALORIE GOAL:

WHAT I ATE:

	Calories	Carbohydrate (45%)	Protein (30%)	Fat (25%)
BREAKFAST				
LUNCH				
DINNER				
SNACK 1				
SNACK 2				

TOTAL CALORIES: **+/- GOAL CALORIES:**

GLASSES OF WATER   ○ ○ ○ ○ ○ ○ ○ ○

WHAT I DID:

	Duration
EXERCISE	

DATE: _____

CALORIE GOAL: _____

WHAT I ATE:

	Calories	Carbohydrate (45%)	Protein (30%)	Fat (25%)
BREAKFAST				
LUNCH				
DINNER				
SNACK 1				
SNACK 2				

TOTAL CALORIES: _____ **+/- GOAL CALORIES:** _____

GLASSES OF WATER ○ ○ ○ ○ ○ ○ ○ ○

WHAT I DID:

	Duration
EXERCISE	

DATE:

CALORIE GOAL:

WHAT I ATE:

		Calories	Carbohydrate (45%)	Protein (30%)	Fat (25%)
BREAKFAST					
LUNCH					
DINNER					
SNACK 1					
SNACK 2					

TOTAL CALORIES:	+/- GOAL CALORIES:
GLASSES OF WATER	○ ○ ○ ○ ○ ○ ○ ○

WHAT I DID:

		Duration
EXERCISE		

DATE:

CALORIE GOAL:

WHAT I ATE:

	Calories	Carbohydrate (45%)	Protein (30%)	Fat (25%)
BREAKFAST				
LUNCH				
DINNER				
SNACK 1				
SNACK 2				

TOTAL CALORIES:	+/- GOAL CALORIES:
GLASSES OF WATER	○ ○ ○ ○ ○ ○ ○ ○

WHAT I DID:

	Duration
EXERCISE	

GRILLED CHICKEN SMOTHERED NACHOS

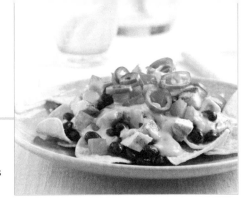

Be sure to wear gloves when working with jalapeño peppers or wash your hands immediately afterward. Though you're sure to love this dish, you won't enjoy it nearly as much if your jalapeño-affected hands make even minimal contact with your eyes!

1	ounce baked tortilla chips (such as Guiltless Gourmet)
¼	cup drained canned 50%-less-sodium black beans, heated
4	ounces grilled extra-lean boneless, skinless chicken breast, cut into small cubes, reheated if necessary
2	tablespoons salsa con queso, all natural if possible (such as Salpica), heated
3	tablespoons finely chopped seeded tomato
2	tablespoons thinly sliced jalapeño chile pepper (wear plastic gloves when handling)

Lay the chips on a dinner plate. Top them evenly with the beans, followed by the chicken. Drizzle the salsa con queso evenly over the top. Top with the tomato and jalapeño pepper slices.

Makes 1 serving

Per serving: 321 calories, 32 g protein, 36 g carbohydrates, 5 g fat (less than 1 g saturated), 65 mg cholesterol, 5 g fiber, 498 mg sodium

DATE:

CALORIE GOAL:

WHAT I ATE:

		Calories	Carbohydrate (45%)	Protein (30%)	Fat (25%)
BREAKFAST					
LUNCH					
DINNER					
SNACK 1					
SNACK 2					

TOTAL CALORIES:	+/- GOAL CALORIES:

GLASSES OF WATER ○ ○ ○ ○ ○ ○ ○ ○

WHAT I DID:

		Duration
EXERCISE		

DATE:

CALORIE GOAL:

WHAT I ATE:

	Calories	Carbohydrate (45%)	Protein (30%)	Fat (25%)
BREAKFAST				
LUNCH				
DINNER				
SNACK 1				
SNACK 2				

TOTAL CALORIES: **+/- GOAL CALORIES:**

GLASSES OF WATER ○ ○ ○ ○ ○ ○ ○ ○

WHAT I DID:

	Duration
EXERCISE	

DATE:

CALORIE GOAL:

WHAT I ATE:

	Calories	Carbohydrate (45%)	Protein (30%)	Fat (25%)
BREAKFAST				
LUNCH				
DINNER				
SNACK 1				
SNACK 2				

TOTAL CALORIES: **+/- GOAL CALORIES:**

GLASSES OF WATER ○ ○ ○ ○ ○ ○ ○ ○

WHAT I DID:

	Duration
EXERCISE	

DATE:

CALORIE GOAL:

WHAT I ATE:

	Calories	Carbohydrate (45%)	Protein (30%)	Fat (25%)
BREAKFAST				
LUNCH				
DINNER				
SNACK 1				
SNACK 2				

TOTAL CALORIES: **+/- GOAL CALORIES:**

GLASSES OF WATER ○ ○ ○ ○ ○ ○ ○ ○

WHAT I DID:

	Duration
EXERCISE	

DATE:

CALORIE GOAL:

WHAT I ATE:

		Calories	Carbohydrate (45%)	Protein (30%)	Fat (25%)
BREAKFAST					
LUNCH					
DINNER					
SNACK 1					
SNACK 2					

TOTAL CALORIES: +/- GOAL CALORIES:

GLASSES OF WATER   ○ , ○ ○ ○ ○ ○ ○ ○

WHAT I DID:

		Duration
EXERCISE		

FRENCH ONION DIP

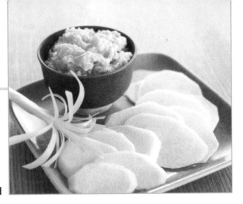

It takes a little time to simmer the onions, but the result is worth waiting for. This tastes just like "the real thing" but has a fraction of the calories.

1	tablespoon olive oil
2¼	pounds yellow onions, peeled, halved vertically, and sliced horizontally into ⅛"-thick half-rounds
1	teaspoon salt
1	teaspoon onion powder
4	ounces low-fat cream cheese, at room temperature
½	cup fat-free Greek-style plain yogurt
2	teaspoons chopped fresh Italian parsley + additional for garnish

In a large skillet or Dutch oven, heat the oil over medium heat. Add the onions and salt. Stir well and cook for 2 to 3 minutes. Continue to simmer, stirring regularly, for 20 to 30 minutes, scraping up any browned bits with a wooden spoon. The onions will be light to medium golden brown (not dark brown) and caramelized. Cool the onions completely.

Place the onions in the bowl of a food processor. Pulse until they're slightly chopped. Remove half of the onions and transfer them to a mixing bowl. To the remaining onions in the food processor, add the onion powder and process until completely pureed. Add the cream cheese and yogurt and process just until smooth. Combine this mixture with the chopped onions and stir well.

Taste and adjust the seasonings as desired, then chill completely. Transfer to a bowl and serve with jicama slices, other veggies, or your favorite baked chips.

Makes 12 (¼-cup) servings

Per serving (¼ cup dip with ½ cup jicama slices): 80 calories, 4 g protein, 10 g carbohydrates, 3 g fat (1 g saturated), 5 mg cholesterol, 2 g fiber, 230 mg sodium

DATE:

CALORIE GOAL:

WHAT I ATE:

	Calories	Carbohydrate (45%)	Protein (30%)	Fat (25%)
BREAKFAST				
LUNCH				
DINNER				
SNACK 1				
SNACK 2				

TOTAL CALORIES: **+/- GOAL CALORIES:**

GLASSES OF WATER   ○ ○ ○ ○ ○ ○ ○ ○

WHAT I DID:

	Duration
EXERCISE	

DATE:

CALORIE GOAL:

WHAT I ATE:

	Calories	Carbohydrate (45%)	Protein (30%)	Fat (25%)
BREAKFAST				
LUNCH				
DINNER				
SNACK 1				
SNACK 2				

TOTAL CALORIES: **+/- GOAL CALORIES:**

GLASSES OF WATER ○ ○ ○ ○ ○ ○ ○ ○

WHAT I DID:

	Duration
EXERCISE	

DATE:

CALORIE GOAL:

WHAT I ATE:

	Calories	Carbohydrate (45%)	Protein (30%)	Fat (25%)
BREAKFAST				
LUNCH				
DINNER				
SNACK 1				
SNACK 2				

TOTAL CALORIES: **+/- GOAL CALORIES:**

GLASSES OF WATER   ○ ○ ○ ○ ○ ○ ○ ○

WHAT I DID:

	Duration
EXERCISE	

DATE:

CALORIE GOAL:

WHAT I ATE:

		Calories	Carbohydrate (45%)	Protein (30%)	Fat (25%)
BREAKFAST					
LUNCH					
DINNER					
SNACK 1					
SNACK 2					

TOTAL CALORIES:	+/- GOAL CALORIES:
GLASSES OF WATER	○ ○ ○ ○ ○ ○ ○ ○

WHAT I DID:

		Duration
EXERCISE		

DATE:

CALORIE GOAL:

WHAT I ATE:

	Calories	Carbohydrate (45%)	Protein (30%)	Fat (25%)
BREAKFAST				
LUNCH				
DINNER				
SNACK 1				
SNACK 2				

TOTAL CALORIES: **+/- GOAL CALORIES:**

GLASSES OF WATER ○ ○ ○ ○ ○ ○ ○ ○

WHAT I DID:

	Duration
EXERCISE	

ROAST BEEF MELT

This satisfying recipe comes from Season 2 contestant Seth Word. If your local supermarket doesn't carry Ezekiel bread, look for a high-fiber multigrain bread.

2	slices Ezekiel bread
2	slices fat-free American cheese
4	ounces lean, thinly sliced deli roast beef
1	tablespoon brown mustard
3	thin slices yellow onion

Top the bread with the cheese and toast it on a grill until the cheese melts. Put the roast beef on the toast. Top with the mustard and onion.

Makes 1 serving

Per serving: 360 calories, 37 g protein, 44 g carbohydrates, 6 g fat (2 g saturated), 40 mg cholesterol, 7 g fiber, 460 mg sodium

Recipe excerpted from *The Biggest Loser: 30-Day Jump Start*

For more ways to live *The Biggest Loser* lifestyle, go to biggestloser.com.

DATE: _____

CALORIE GOAL: _____

WHAT I ATE:

		Calories	Carbohydrate (45%)	Protein (30%)	Fat (25%)
BREAKFAST					
LUNCH					
DINNER					
SNACK 1					
SNACK 2					

TOTAL CALORIES: _____   **+/- GOAL CALORIES:** _____

GLASSES OF WATER ○ ○ ○ ○ ○ ○ ○ ○

WHAT I DID:

		Duration
EXERCISE		

DATE:

CALORIE GOAL:

WHAT I ATE:

	Calories	Carbohydrate (45%)	Protein (30%)	Fat (25%)
BREAKFAST				
LUNCH				
DINNER				
SNACK 1				
SNACK 2				

TOTAL CALORIES: **+/- GOAL CALORIES:**

GLASSES OF WATER ○ ○ ○ ○ ○ ○ ○ ○

WHAT I DID:

	Duration
EXERCISE	

DATE:

CALORIE GOAL:

WHAT I ATE:

	Calories	Carbohydrate (45%)	Protein (30%)	Fat (25%)
BREAKFAST				
LUNCH				
DINNER				
SNACK 1				
SNACK 2				

TOTAL CALORIES: **+/- GOAL CALORIES:**

GLASSES OF WATER   ○ ○ ○ ○ ○ ○ ○ ○

WHAT I DID:

	Duration
EXERCISE	

DATE: _____

CALORIE GOAL: _____

WHAT I ATE:

		Calories	Carbohydrate (45%)	Protein (30%)	Fat (25%)
BREAKFAST					
LUNCH					
DINNER					
SNACK 1					
SNACK 2					

TOTAL CALORIES: _____ **+/- GOAL CALORIES:** _____

GLASSES OF WATER ○ ○ ○ ○ ○ ○ ○ ○

WHAT I DID:

		Duration
EXERCISE		

DATE:

CALORIE GOAL:

WHAT I ATE:

	Calories	Carbohydrate (45%)	Protein (30%)	Fat (25%)
BREAKFAST				
LUNCH				
DINNER				
SNACK 1				
SNACK 2				

TOTAL CALORIES:　　　　　**+/- GOAL CALORIES:**

GLASSES OF WATER　○　○　○　○　○　○　○　○

WHAT I DID:

	Duration
EXERCISE	

OUT-TO-LUNCH TOSTADA SALAD

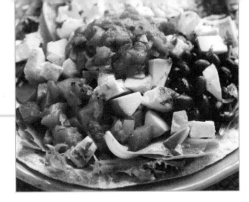

This salad is a healthier rendition of one of the contestants' favorite dishes from a Mexican restaurant near the Ranch. It's loaded with fiber and protein and is very filling.

1	whole wheat tortilla
2	cups baby lettuce mix
¼	cup cooked brown rice
¼	cup cooked black beans
½	cup fire-roasted sliced bell peppers, diced
4	ounces grilled chicken breast, diced
¼	avocado, diced
½	cup low-sodium salsa
1	tablespoon fat-free Greek-style plain yogurt
2	tablespoons chopped cilantro

Toast the tortilla in a toaster oven until crisp. Place the lettuce mix on the tortilla. Then, in clockwise fashion, top the lettuce with the rice, beans, and bell peppers. Sprinkle the chicken and avocado on top. Place a spoonful of salsa in the center and top with a dollop of yogurt. Garnish with the cilantro.

Makes 1 serving

Per serving: 400 calories, 39 g protein, 44 g carbohydrates, 11 g fat (9 g saturated), 65 mg cholesterol, 18 g fiber, 310 mg sodium

DATE:

CALORIE GOAL:

WHAT I ATE:

	Calories	Carbohydrate (45%)	Protein (30%)	Fat (25%)
BREAKFAST				
LUNCH				
DINNER				
SNACK 1				
SNACK 2				

TOTAL CALORIES: +/- GOAL CALORIES:

GLASSES OF WATER   ○ ○ ○ ○ ○ ○ ○ ○

WHAT I DID:

	Duration
EXERCISE	

DATE:

CALORIE GOAL:

WHAT I ATE:

		Calories	Carbohydrate (45%)	Protein (30%)	Fat (25%)
BREAKFAST					
LUNCH					
DINNER					
SNACK 1					
SNACK 2					

TOTAL CALORIES: **+/- GOAL CALORIES:**

GLASSES OF WATER ○ ○ ○ ○ ○ ○ ○ ○

WHAT I DID:

		Duration
EXERCISE		

DATE:

CALORIE GOAL:

WHAT I ATE:

		Calories	Carbohydrate (45%)	Protein (30%)	Fat (25%)
BREAKFAST					
LUNCH					
DINNER					
SNACK 1					
SNACK 2					

TOTAL CALORIES: **+/- GOAL CALORIES:**

GLASSES OF WATER   ○ ○ ○ ○ ○ ○ ○ ○

WHAT I DID:

		Duration
EXERCISE		

DATE:

CALORIE GOAL:

WHAT I ATE:

	Calories	Carbohydrate (45%)	Protein (30%)	Fat (25%)
BREAKFAST				
LUNCH				
DINNER				
SNACK 1				
SNACK 2				

TOTAL CALORIES: +/- GOAL CALORIES:

GLASSES OF WATER ○ ○ ○ ○ ○ ○ ○ ○

WHAT I DID:

	Duration
EXERCISE	

DATE: | CALORIE GOAL:

WHAT I ATE:

	Calories	Carbohydrate (45%)	Protein (30%)	Fat (25%)
BREAKFAST				
LUNCH				
DINNER				
SNACK 1				
SNACK 2				

TOTAL CALORIES: **+/- GOAL CALORIES:**

GLASSES OF WATER ○ ○ ○ ○ ○ ○ ○ ○

WHAT I DID:

	Duration
EXERCISE	

BELL PEPPER–CHICKEN SANDWICH

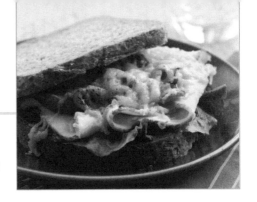

Season 7's Estella Hayes helped invent this recipe one day at the Ranch. The addition of bell peppers gives this chicken sandwich added flavor, and the sprouted grain bread lends a great texture.

1	tablespoon yellow or spicy mustard
2	slices sprouted whole grain bread (Trader Joe's or other brand), toasted
1	large leaf romaine lettuce
3	ounces lean, low-sodium sliced chicken breast
½	roasted red bell pepper, cut in strips
¼	cup shredded reduced-fat Mexican four-cheese blend

Spread the mustard on 1 piece of toast. Top with the lettuce, chicken, and bell pepper, and end with the cheese.

Place the half sandwich under a broiler or in a toaster oven for 20 to 30 seconds, until the cheese melts. Top with the second piece of toast. Cut in half. Serve immediately.

Makes 1 serving

Per serving: 310 calories, 31 g protein, 30 g carbohydrates, 7 g fat (3 g saturated), 65 mg cholesterol, 6 g fiber, 1,380 mg sodium

DATE:

CALORIE GOAL:

WHAT I ATE:

	Calories	Carbohydrate (45%)	Protein (30%)	Fat (25%)
BREAKFAST				
LUNCH				
DINNER				
SNACK 1				
SNACK 2				

TOTAL CALORIES: **+/- GOAL CALORIES:**

GLASSES OF WATER ○ ○ ○ ○ ○ ○ ○ ○

WHAT I DID:

	Duration
EXERCISE	

DATE: _____

CALORIE GOAL: _____

WHAT I ATE:

	Calories	Carbohydrate (45%)	Protein (30%)	Fat (25%)
BREAKFAST				
LUNCH				
DINNER				
SNACK 1				
SNACK 2				

TOTAL CALORIES: _____ **+/- GOAL CALORIES:** _____

GLASSES OF WATER ○ ○ ○ ○ ○ ○ ○ ○

WHAT I DID:

	Duration
EXERCISE	

DATE: _____

CALORIE GOAL: _____

WHAT I ATE:

		Calories	Carbohydrate (45%)	Protein (30%)	Fat (25%)
BREAKFAST					
LUNCH					
DINNER					
SNACK 1					
SNACK 2					

TOTAL CALORIES:	+/- GOAL CALORIES:

GLASSES OF WATER ○ ○ ○ ○ ○ ○ ○ ○

WHAT I DID:

	Duration
EXERCISE	

DATE: _____

CALORIE GOAL: _____

WHAT I ATE:

		Calories	Carbohydrate (45%)	Protein (30%)	Fat (25%)
BREAKFAST					
LUNCH					
DINNER					
SNACK 1					
SNACK 2					

TOTAL CALORIES: _____ **+/- GOAL CALORIES:** _____

GLASSES OF WATER ○ ○ ○ ○ ○ ○ ○ ○

WHAT I DID:

	Duration
EXERCISE	

DATE: _____

CALORIE GOAL: _____

WHAT I ATE:

	Calories	Carbohydrate (45%)	Protein (30%)	Fat (25%)
BREAKFAST				
LUNCH				
DINNER				
SNACK 1				
SNACK 2				

TOTAL CALORIES: _____ **+/- GOAL CALORIES:** _____

GLASSES OF WATER ○ ○ ○ ○ ○ ○ ○ ○

WHAT I DID:

	Duration
EXERCISE	

FIRE-ROASTED TOMATO SOUP

America's all-time favorite comfort soup is jazzed up with the addition of flavorful fire-roasted tomatoes and aromatic, spicy ginger.

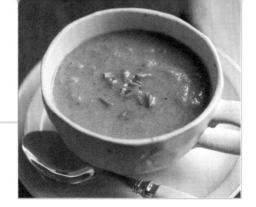

1	teaspoon olive oil
2	tablespoons minced shallot or onion
4	quarter-size slices peeled fresh ginger
1	tablespoon chopped garlic
1½	cups (14½-ounce can) diced fire-roasted tomatoes
1	cup fat-free chicken broth or vegetable broth
½	cup 1% or fat-free milk
	Salt and pepper to taste
1	tablespoon chopped fresh chives or scallion

In a 2-quart saucepan, heat the oil over medium heat. Add the shallot and ginger and cook until softened, about 1 minute.

Add the garlic and tomatoes to the saucepan. Simmer for about 4 minutes, until the mixture begins to thicken. Add the broth and milk and just bring to a boil.

Carefully transfer the soup to a food processor or blender. Process or blend until smooth. Return to the saucepan and serve immediately. Add salt and pepper and garnish with the chives or scallion.

Makes 4 (¾-cup) servings, or 3 cups

Per serving: 60 calories, 2 g protein, 8 g carbohydrates, 2 g fat (0 g saturated), 0 mg cholesterol, 2 g fiber, 360 mg sodium

DATE:

CALORIE GOAL:

WHAT I ATE:

	Calories	Carbohydrate (45%)	Protein (30%)	Fat (25%)
BREAKFAST				
LUNCH				
DINNER				
SNACK 1				
SNACK 2				

TOTAL CALORIES: **+/- GOAL CALORIES:**

GLASSES OF WATER   ○ ○ ○ ○ ○ ○ ○ ○

WHAT I DID:

	Duration
EXERCISE	

DATE:

CALORIE GOAL:

WHAT I ATE:

		Calories	Carbohydrate (45%)	Protein (30%)	Fat (25%)
BREAKFAST					
LUNCH					
DINNER					
SNACK 1					
SNACK 2					

TOTAL CALORIES: **+/- GOAL CALORIES:**

GLASSES OF WATER ○ ○ ○ ○ ○ ○ ○ ○

WHAT I DID:

		Duration
EXERCISE		

DATE:

CALORIE GOAL:

WHAT I ATE:

		Calories	Carbohydrate (45%)	Protein (30%)	Fat (25%)
BREAKFAST					
LUNCH					
DINNER					
SNACK 1					
SNACK 2					

TOTAL CALORIES: **+/- GOAL CALORIES:**

GLASSES OF WATER ○ ○ ○ ○ ○ ○ ○ ○

WHAT I DID:

		Duration
EXERCISE		

DATE:

CALORIE GOAL:

WHAT I ATE:

	Calories	Carbohydrate (45%)	Protein (30%)	Fat (25%)
BREAKFAST				
LUNCH				
DINNER				
SNACK 1				
SNACK 2				

TOTAL CALORIES: **+/- GOAL CALORIES:**

GLASSES OF WATER ○ ○ ○ ○ ○ ○ ○ ○

WHAT I DID:

	Duration
EXERCISE	

DATE: _____

CALORIE GOAL: _____

WHAT I ATE:

		Calories	Carbohydrate (45%)	Protein (30%)	Fat (25%)
BREAKFAST					
LUNCH					
DINNER					
SNACK 1					
SNACK 2					

TOTAL CALORIES: _____ **+/- GOAL CALORIES:** _____

GLASSES OF WATER ○ ○ ○ ○ ○ ○ ○ ○

WHAT I DID:

		Duration
EXERCISE		

BLACK BEAN QUESADILLAS

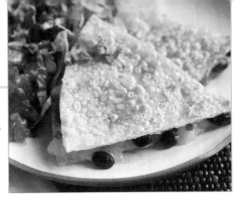

This is one of Season 8 winner Danny Cahill's favorite meals, especially since it's what his wife, Darci, prepared for him the first day he came home from the Ranch. The beans, salsa, and cheese give these quesadillas all the flavor and texture you crave from rich Mexican food, with only 6 grams of fat per serving.

2	brown rice tortillas (burrito size)
2	slices reduced-fat pepper Jack cheese
½	cup black beans
¼	cup fresh salsa
2	cups shredded romaine lettuce

Coat a large nonstick skillet with cooking spray and heat over medium heat.

One at a time, warm each tortilla on both sides. Leave the second tortilla in the skillet and tear the cheese into pieces to cover the tortilla in a single layer. Spread the beans over the tortilla and heat for 1 to 2 minutes. Add the second tortilla and heat for 1 minute longer. Turn the quesadilla over and heat until the cheese is just melted.

Remove the quesadilla from the pan and cut into 6 triangles. Place 3 triangles on each of 2 plates and top with salsa and lettuce.

Makes 2 servings

Per serving: 240 calories, 10 g protein, 38 g carbohydrates, 6 g fat (2 g saturated), 10 mg cholesterol, 7 g fiber, 290 mg sodium

DATE: _____

CALORIE GOAL: _____

WHAT I ATE:

		Calories	Carbohydrate (45%)	Protein (30%)	Fat (25%)
BREAKFAST					
LUNCH					
DINNER					
SNACK 1					
SNACK 2					

TOTAL CALORIES: _____ **+/- GOAL CALORIES:** _____

GLASSES OF WATER ○ ○ ○ ○ ○ ○ ○ ○

WHAT I DID:

		Duration
EXERCISE		

DATE:

CALORIE GOAL:

WHAT I ATE:

	Calories	Carbohydrate (45%)	Protein (30%)	Fat (25%)
BREAKFAST				
LUNCH				
DINNER				
SNACK 1				
SNACK 2				

TOTAL CALORIES: **+/- GOAL CALORIES:**

GLASSES OF WATER ○ ○ ○ ○ ○ ○ ○ ○

WHAT I DID:

	Duration
EXERCISE	

DATE:

CALORIE GOAL:

WHAT I ATE:

	Calories	Carbohydrate (45%)	Protein (30%)	Fat (25%)
BREAKFAST				
LUNCH				
DINNER				
SNACK 1				
SNACK 2				

TOTAL CALORIES: **+/- GOAL CALORIES:**

GLASSES OF WATER ○ ○ ○ ○ ○ ○ ○ ○

WHAT I DID:

	Duration
EXERCISE	

DATE:

CALORIE GOAL:

WHAT I ATE:

	Calories	Carbohydrate (45%)	Protein (30%)	Fat (25%)
BREAKFAST				
LUNCH				
DINNER				
SNACK 1				
SNACK 2				

TOTAL CALORIES: **+/- GOAL CALORIES:**

GLASSES OF WATER ○ ○ ○ ○ ○ ○ ○ ○

WHAT I DID:

	Duration
EXERCISE	

DATE: _____   **CALORIE GOAL:** _____

WHAT I ATE:

		Calories	Carbohydrate (45%)	Protein (30%)	Fat (25%)
BREAKFAST					
LUNCH					
DINNER					
SNACK 1					
SNACK 2					

TOTAL CALORIES:	**+/- GOAL CALORIES:**

GLASSES OF WATER ○ ○ ○ ○ ○ ○ ○ ○

WHAT I DID:

		Duration
EXERCISE		

APPLE COBBLER

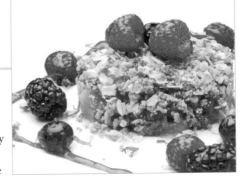

What could be more satisfying than a steaming bowl of apple cobbler, complete with a sweet, crumbly topping? Guests at *The Biggest Loser* Resort at Fitness Ridge enjoy this delicious, fruity dessert after a long day of sweating it out in the gym. At just 155 calories per serving, this is one treat anyone can fit into their calorie budget.

4 cups peeled and sliced apples

⅛ cup maple syrup

1 tablespoon cinnamon

3 tablespoons cane sugar

¼ cup instant oats plus ½ cup

¼ cup pecans

1 tablespoon soy butter

1 teaspoon cinnamon

3 tablespoon cane sugar

Preheat the oven to 350°F.

Spray a 9 x 9 pan with nonstick cooking spray. Layer the apples on the bottom of the pan. Then drizzle the maple syrup over the fruit and sprinkle the cinnamon and cane sugar.

In a food processor, combine the ¼ cup instant oats, pecans, soy butter, cinnamon, and cane sugar. Blend until all lumps are gone and everything is evenly chopped. Pour into a mixing bowl. Add the remaining ½ cup of instant oats to the bowl and mix together. Sprinkle the mixture over the fruit and bake for an hour or until the fruit sets up. Cool for 15 minutes and serve.

Makes 9 servings

Per serving: 155 calories, 4 g protein, 27 grams carbohydrates, 6 g fat (0 g saturated), 0 mg cholesterol, 4 g fiber, 12 mg sodium

For more ways to live *The Biggest Loser* lifestyle, go to biggestloser.com.

DATE: _____

CALORIE GOAL: _____

WHAT I ATE:

	Calories	Carbohydrate (45%)	Protein (30%)	Fat (25%)
BREAKFAST				
LUNCH				
DINNER				
SNACK 1				
SNACK 2				

TOTAL CALORIES: _____ +/- GOAL CALORIES: _____

GLASSES OF WATER ◯ ◯ ◯ ◯ ◯ ◯ ◯ ◯

WHAT I DID:

	Duration
EXERCISE	

DATE:

CALORIE GOAL:

WHAT I ATE:

		Calories	Carbohydrate (45%)	Protein (30%)	Fat (25%)
BREAKFAST					
LUNCH					
DINNER					
SNACK 1					
SNACK 2					

TOTAL CALORIES:	+/- GOAL CALORIES:
GLASSES OF WATER	○ ○ ○ ○ ○ ○ ○ ○

WHAT I DID:

		Duration
EXERCISE		

DATE: _____

CALORIE GOAL: _____

WHAT I ATE:

		Calories	Carbohydrate (45%)	Protein (30%)	Fat (25%)
BREAKFAST					
LUNCH					
DINNER					
SNACK 1					
SNACK 2					

TOTAL CALORIES:	+/- GOAL CALORIES:

GLASSES OF WATER ○ ○ ○ ○ ○ ○ ○ ○

WHAT I DID:

		Duration
EXERCISE		

DATE:

CALORIE GOAL:

WHAT I ATE:

	Calories	Carbohydrate (45%)	Protein (30%)	Fat (25%)
BREAKFAST				
LUNCH				
DINNER				
SNACK 1				
SNACK 2				

TOTAL CALORIES: **+/- GOAL CALORIES:**

GLASSES OF WATER ○ ○ ○ ○ ○ ○ ○ ○

WHAT I DID:

	Duration
EXERCISE	

DATE: _____

CALORIE GOAL: _____

WHAT I ATE:

		Calories	Carbohydrate (45%)	Protein (30%)	Fat (25%)
BREAKFAST					
LUNCH					
DINNER					
SNACK 1					
SNACK 2					

TOTAL CALORIES: _____   **+/- GOAL CALORIES:** _____

GLASSES OF WATER ○ ○ ○ ○ ○ ○ ○ ○

WHAT I DID:

		Duration
EXERCISE		

TODAY'S TUNA SANDWICHES

People often order tuna sandwiches thinking that they're healthy. Well . . . the tuna is, but until you've made tuna salad yourself a number of times, you have no idea how much mayo can be packed into a small serving. This recipe gives you the taste you love with a fraction of the fat and calories contained in traditional tuna salad.

2	(6-ounce) cans chunk light tuna in water, drained
3	tablespoons low-fat mayonnaise
¼	cup finely chopped celery
¼	cup finely chopped red onion
	Ground black pepper to taste
8	slices sesame sprouted grain bread or whole grain bread (such as Ezekiel 4:9 brand)
16	thin slices tomato
16	thin slices cucumber
1⅓	cups alfalfa sprouts

In a medium bowl, mix the tuna with the mayonnaise until well combined. Stir in the celery and onion and season with pepper.

Place 1 piece of bread on each of 4 serving plates. Evenly place 4 slices of tomato, followed by 4 slices of cucumber, on each bread slice. Top each with one-fourth of the tuna mixture (about ¼ cup + 2 tablespoons each), followed by one-fourth of the alfalfa sprouts. Top each sandwich with a remaining bread slice.

Makes 4 servings

Per serving: 284 calories, 27 g protein, 34 g carbohydrates, 3 g fat (trace saturated), 21 mg cholesterol, 7 g fiber, 410 mg sodium

DATE:

CALORIE GOAL:

WHAT I ATE:

	Calories	Carbohydrate (45%)	Protein (30%)	Fat (25%)
BREAKFAST				
LUNCH				
DINNER				
SNACK 1				
SNACK 2				

TOTAL CALORIES: **+/- GOAL CALORIES:**

GLASSES OF WATER ○ ○ ○ ○ ○ ○ ○ ○

WHAT I DID:

	Duration
EXERCISE	

DATE:

CALORIE GOAL:

WHAT I ATE:

		Calories	Carbohydrate (45%)	Protein (30%)	Fat (25%)
BREAKFAST					
LUNCH					
DINNER					
SNACK 1					
SNACK 2					

TOTAL CALORIES: **+/- GOAL CALORIES:**

GLASSES OF WATER ○ ○ ○ ○ ○ ○ ○ ○

WHAT I DID:

		Duration
EXERCISE		

DATE:

CALORIE GOAL:

WHAT I ATE:

	Calories	Carbohydrate (45%)	Protein (30%)	Fat (25%)
BREAKFAST				
LUNCH				
DINNER				
SNACK 1				
SNACK 2				

TOTAL CALORIES: **+/- GOAL CALORIES:**

GLASSES OF WATER   ○ ○ ○ ○ ○ ○ ○ ○

WHAT I DID:

	Duration
EXERCISE	

DATE:

CALORIE GOAL:

WHAT I ATE:

		Calories	Carbohydrate (45%)	Protein (30%)	Fat (25%)
BREAKFAST					
LUNCH					
DINNER					
SNACK 1					
SNACK 2					

TOTAL CALORIES: **+/- GOAL CALORIES:**

GLASSES OF WATER ○ ○ ○ ○ ○ ○ ○ ○

WHAT I DID:

		Duration
EXERCISE		

DATE:

CALORIE GOAL:

WHAT I ATE:

	Calories	Carbohydrate (45%)	Protein (30%)	Fat (25%)
BREAKFAST				
LUNCH				
DINNER				
SNACK 1				
SNACK 2				

TOTAL CALORIES:	+/- GOAL CALORIES:

GLASSES OF WATER	○ ○ ○ ○ ○ ○ ○ ○

WHAT I DID:

	Duration
EXERCISE	

CHICKEN SALAD DIJON WITH GRAPES AND APPLE

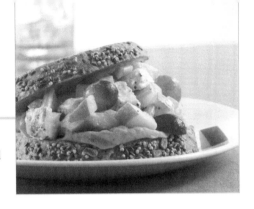

Dijon mustard fans will love this twist on traditional chicken salad—and will be shocked by the creaminess of the dressing, given that it has about one-third of the calories and one-fourth of the fat found in most chicken salads.

Serve over a bed of butter lettuce or fresh spinach or on sprouted grain or multigrain bread.

1	pound trimmed boneless, skinless chicken breasts
3	teaspoons extra-virgin olive oil
	Salt and pepper to taste
3	tablespoons plain fat-free yogurt
3	tablespoons Dijon mustard
⅓	cup chopped celery
⅓	cup seedless grapes, halved
⅓	cup chopped red apple

Preheat a grill to high heat.

Rub the chicken all over with 1 teaspoon of the oil and season with salt and pepper. Place on the grill and cook for 3 to 5 minutes per side, or until the chicken is no longer pink and the juices run clear. Allow the chicken to cool, then cut it into bite-size cubes.

In a large mixing bowl, whisk together the yogurt, mustard, and remaining 2 teaspoons oil. Add the chicken, celery, grapes, and apple. Gently toss to combine. Season as desired.

Makes 4 servings

Per serving: 173 calories, 27 g protein, 4 g carbohydrates, 5 g fat (less than 1 g saturated), 66 mg cholesterol, trace fiber, 361 mg sodium

DATE:

CALORIE GOAL:

WHAT I ATE:

		Calories	Carbohydrate (45%)	Protein (30%)	Fat (25%)
BREAKFAST					
LUNCH					
DINNER					
SNACK 1					
SNACK 2					

TOTAL CALORIES:	+/- GOAL CALORIES:
GLASSES OF WATER	○ ○ ○ ○ ○ ○ ○ ○

WHAT I DID:

	Duration
EXERCISE	

DATE:

CALORIE GOAL:

WHAT I ATE:

	Calories	Carbohydrate (45%)	Protein (30%)	Fat (25%)
BREAKFAST				
LUNCH				
DINNER				
SNACK 1				
SNACK 2				

TOTAL CALORIES: **+/- GOAL CALORIES:**

GLASSES OF WATER   ○ ○ ○ ○ ○ ○ ○ ○

WHAT I DID:

	Duration
EXERCISE	

DATE:

CALORIE GOAL:

WHAT I ATE:

	Calories	Carbohydrate (45%)	Protein (30%)	Fat (25%)
BREAKFAST				
LUNCH				
DINNER				
SNACK 1				
SNACK 2				

TOTAL CALORIES:	+/- GOAL CALORIES:

GLASSES OF WATER ○ ○ ○ ○ ○ ○ ○ ○

WHAT I DID:

	Duration
EXERCISE	

DATE:

CALORIE GOAL:

WHAT I ATE:

		Calories	Carbohydrate (45%)	Protein (30%)	Fat (25%)
BREAKFAST					
LUNCH					
DINNER					
SNACK 1					
SNACK 2					

TOTAL CALORIES: **+/- GOAL CALORIES:**

GLASSES OF WATER ○ ○ ○ ○ ○ ○ ○ ○

WHAT I DID:

		Duration
EXERCISE		

DATE:

CALORIE GOAL:

WHAT I ATE:

	Calories	Carbohydrate (45%)	Protein (30%)	Fat (25%)
BREAKFAST				
LUNCH				
DINNER				
SNACK 1				
SNACK 2				

TOTAL CALORIES: +/- GOAL CALORIES:

GLASSES OF WATER   ○ ○ ○ ○ ○ ○ ○ ○

WHAT I DID:

	Duration
EXERCISE	

GRILLED SALMON BURGERS

These burgers are a delicious way to enjoy omega-3-rich fish. If you don't have a grill, they can also be cooked in a large nonstick skillet over medium-high heat.

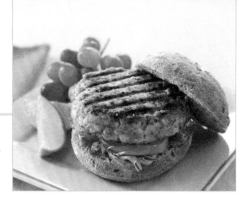

1 pound skinless salmon fillet, cut into 1" cubes

1 tablespoon Dijon mustard

1 tablespoon grated lime peel

1 tablespoon peeled, minced fresh ginger

1 tablespoon chopped cilantro

1 teaspoon reduced-sodium soy sauce

½ teaspoon ground coriander

Salt and pepper to taste

Fresh lime wedges

Cilantro leaves

Preheat the barbecue grill to medium-high heat. Lightly coat the grill rack with olive oil cooking spray.

In a food processor, pulse the salmon just enough to grind it coarsely. Transfer the salmon to a large bowl and mix in the mustard, lime peel, ginger, cilantro, soy sauce, and coriander. Form the salmon into 4 patties and season with salt and pepper. Grill the burgers or cook them in a skillet, turning once, until done, 4 minutes per side for medium.

Garnish with fresh lime wedges and cilantro leaves.

Makes 4 servings

Per serving: 170 calories, 23 g protein, 1 g carbohydrates, 7 g fat (1 g saturated), 60 mg cholesterol, 0 g fiber, 150 mg sodium

DATE:

CALORIE GOAL:

WHAT I ATE:

	Calories	Carbohydrate (45%)	Protein (30%)	Fat (25%)
BREAKFAST				
LUNCH				
DINNER				
SNACK 1				
SNACK 2				

TOTAL CALORIES: **+/- GOAL CALORIES:**

GLASSES OF WATER   ○ ○ ○ ○ ○ ○ ○ ○

WHAT I DID:

	Duration
EXERCISE	

DATE:

CALORIE GOAL:

WHAT I ATE:

		Calories	Carbohydrate (45%)	Protein (30%)	Fat (25%)
BREAKFAST					
LUNCH					
DINNER					
SNACK 1					
SNACK 2					

TOTAL CALORIES:	+/- GOAL CALORIES:

GLASSES OF WATER	○ ○ ○ ○ ○ ○ ○ ○

WHAT I DID:

		Duration
EXERCISE		

DATE:

CALORIE GOAL:

WHAT I ATE:

	Calories	Carbohydrate (45%)	Protein (30%)	Fat (25%)
BREAKFAST				
LUNCH				
DINNER				
SNACK 1				
SNACK 2				

TOTAL CALORIES: **+/- GOAL CALORIES:**

GLASSES OF WATER   ○ ○ ○ ○ ○ ○ ○ ○

WHAT I DID:

	Duration
EXERCISE	

DATE:

CALORIE GOAL:

WHAT I ATE:

	Calories	Carbohydrate (45%)	Protein (30%)	Fat (25%)
BREAKFAST				
LUNCH				
DINNER				
SNACK 1				
SNACK 2				

TOTAL CALORIES:	+/- GOAL CALORIES:

GLASSES OF WATER ○ ○ ○ ○ ○ ○ ○ ○

WHAT I DID:

	Duration
EXERCISE	

DATE:

CALORIE GOAL:

WHAT I ATE:

	Calories	Carbohydrate (45%)	Protein (30%)	Fat (25%)
BREAKFAST				
LUNCH				
DINNER				
SNACK 1				
SNACK 2				

TOTAL CALORIES: **+/- GOAL CALORIES:**

GLASSES OF WATER ○ ○ ○ ○ ○ ○ ○ ○

WHAT I DID:

	Duration
EXERCISE	

RANCH-STYLE "SPAGHETTI" MARINARA

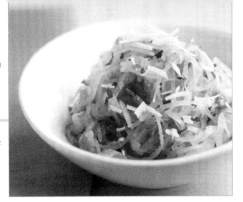

This flavorful squash can always be found in the kitchen at the Ranch as a creative replacement for white pasta. Add turkey meatballs and a salad, and you have a meal.

1	medium spaghetti squash (about 1½ pounds), washed, halved lengthwise, and seeds removed
2	cups low-fat marinara sauce
2	tablespoons chopped fresh basil or parsley
2	tablespoons grated Parmesan or Romano cheese

Preheat the oven to 375°F. Lightly coat a baking sheet with olive oil cooking spray.

Pierce the outside of each half of the squash a few times with a fork. Place the squash cut side down on the baking sheet and bake for about 45 minutes, until very tender when tested with a fork. Allow to cool slightly.

While the squash is baking, warm the marinara sauce.

Using the tines of a fork, rake the spaghetti-like threads of the squash into a mixing bowl. (There will be about 3 cups.) Discard the skin. Pour the hot marinara sauce over the squash and toss gently. Garnish with the basil or parsley and cheese.

Makes 6 servings

Per serving: 130 calories, 4 g protein, 21 g carbohydrates, 3 g fat (1 g saturated), 5 mg cholesterol, 2 g fiber, 280 mg sodium

DATE:

CALORIE GOAL:

WHAT I ATE:

	Calories	Carbohydrate (45%)	Protein (30%)	Fat (25%)
BREAKFAST				
LUNCH				
DINNER				
SNACK 1				
SNACK 2				

TOTAL CALORIES: **+/- GOAL CALORIES:**

GLASSES OF WATER   ○ ○ ○ ○ ○ ○ ○ ○

WHAT I DID:

	Duration
EXERCISE	

DATE:

CALORIE GOAL:

WHAT I ATE:

	Calories	Carbohydrate (45%)	Protein (30%)	Fat (25%)
BREAKFAST				
LUNCH				
DINNER				
SNACK 1				
SNACK 2				

TOTAL CALORIES: **+/- GOAL CALORIES:**

GLASSES OF WATER ○ ○ ○ ○ ○ ○ ○ ○

WHAT I DID:

	Duration
EXERCISE	

DATE:

CALORIE GOAL:

WHAT I ATE:

	Calories	Carbohydrate (45%)	Protein (30%)	Fat (25%)
BREAKFAST				
LUNCH				
DINNER				
SNACK 1				
SNACK 2				

TOTAL CALORIES:	+/- GOAL CALORIES:

GLASSES OF WATER ○ ○ ○ ○ ○ ○ ○ ○

WHAT I DID:

	Duration
EXERCISE	

DATE:

CALORIE GOAL:

WHAT I ATE:

	Calories	Carbohydrate (45%)	Protein (30%)	Fat (25%)
BREAKFAST				
LUNCH				
DINNER				
SNACK 1				
SNACK 2				

TOTAL CALORIES: **+/- GOAL CALORIES:**

GLASSES OF WATER ○ ○ ○ ○ ○ ○ ○ ○

WHAT I DID:

	Duration
EXERCISE	

DATE: _____

CALORIE GOAL: _____

WHAT I ATE:

		Calories	Carbohydrate (45%)	Protein (30%)	Fat (25%)
BREAKFAST					
LUNCH					
DINNER					
SNACK 1					
SNACK 2					

TOTAL CALORIES: _____ **+/- GOAL CALORIES:** _____

GLASSES OF WATER ○ ○ ○ ○ ○ ○ ○ ○

WHAT I DID:

	Duration
EXERCISE	

DOC'S CHILI

A simmering pot of Doc's Chili could be found on the Ranch stove every week during Season 2. This crowd-pleasing favorite is short on preparation time and long on flavor.

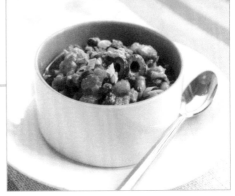

3	cups chopped yellow onions
1¼	pounds 99% lean ground turkey or lean turkey sausage
3	cups diced tomatoes or 1 can (28 ounces) roasted diced tomatoes, undrained
1½	cups cooked pinto beans or 1 can (15 ounces) pinto beans, rinsed and drained
1½	cups cooked black beans or 1 can (15 ounces) black beans, rinsed and drained
1	cup fat-free, low-sodium chicken broth
2	tablespoons chopped garlic
2	tablespoons chili powder
1	tablespoon chopped fresh oregano or 1 teaspoon dried
1	teaspoon ground cumin
1	teaspoon mustard powder
½	cup sliced black olives
½	cup chopped scallions or chopped cilantro

Coat a large saucepan or Dutch oven with olive oil cooking spray. Add the onions and cook over medium-high heat until soft. Add the ground turkey and cook for about 6 minutes, or until no longer pink. Add the tomatoes, pinto and black beans, broth, garlic, chili powder, oregano, cumin, and mustard powder. Bring to a boil over high heat, then reduce to low. Cover and simmer for 20 minutes.

Garnish with the olives and scallions or cilantro.

Makes 12 (1-cup) servings

Per serving: 150 calories, 16 g protein, 17 g carbohydrates, 2 g fat (0 g saturated), 20 mg cholesterol, 5 g fiber, 150 mg sodium

DATE:

CALORIE GOAL:

WHAT I ATE:

	Calories	Carbohydrate (45%)	Protein (30%)	Fat (25%)
BREAKFAST				
LUNCH				
DINNER				
SNACK 1				
SNACK 2				

TOTAL CALORIES: **+/- GOAL CALORIES:**

GLASSES OF WATER ○ ○ ○ ○ ○ ○ ○ ○

WHAT I DID:

	Duration
EXERCISE	

DATE:

CALORIE GOAL:

WHAT I ATE:

		Calories	Carbohydrate (45%)	Protein (30%)	Fat (25%)
BREAKFAST					
LUNCH					
DINNER					
SNACK 1					
SNACK 2					

TOTAL CALORIES: **+/- GOAL CALORIES:**

GLASSES OF WATER ○ ○ ○ ○ ○ ○ ○ ○

WHAT I DID:

		Duration
EXERCISE		

DATE:

CALORIE GOAL:

WHAT I ATE:

		Calories	Carbohydrate (45%)	Protein (30%)	Fat (25%)
BREAKFAST					
LUNCH					
DINNER					
SNACK 1					
SNACK 2					

TOTAL CALORIES: **+/- GOAL CALORIES:**

GLASSES OF WATER ○ ○ ○ ○ ○ ○ ○ ○

WHAT I DID:

		Duration
EXERCISE		

DATE:

CALORIE GOAL:

WHAT I ATE:

	Calories	Carbohydrate (45%)	Protein (30%)	Fat (25%)
BREAKFAST				
LUNCH				
DINNER				
SNACK 1				
SNACK 2				

TOTAL CALORIES: **+/- GOAL CALORIES:**

GLASSES OF WATER ○ ○ ○ ○ ○ ○ ○ ○

WHAT I DID:

	Duration
EXERCISE	

DATE: _____

CALORIE GOAL: _____

WHAT I ATE:

		Calories	Carbohydrate (45%)	Protein (30%)	Fat (25%)
BREAKFAST					
LUNCH					
DINNER					
SNACK 1					
SNACK 2					

TOTAL CALORIES: _____ **+/- GOAL CALORIES:** _____

GLASSES OF WATER ○ ○ ○ ○ ○ ○ ○ ○

WHAT I DID:

		Duration
EXERCISE		

GRILLED TURKEY CUTLETS WITH SALSA

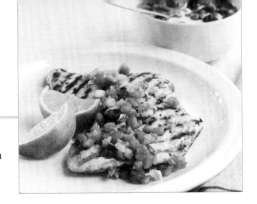

Turkey cutlets cook quickly and much more evenly than larger cuts of turkey. This dish can be made with any kind of salsa you'd like, so you won't grow tired of the same old recipe.

1	teaspoon extra-virgin olive oil
1	pound boneless, skinless turkey cutlets
⅛	to ¼ teaspoon seasoned salt, to taste
½	teaspoon salt-free, extra-spicy seasoning (such as Mrs. Dash Extra Spicy)
6	tablespoons fresh salsa (refrigerated, not jarred), any variety

Preheat a grill to high heat.

Rub the oil all over the cutlets and season evenly with the seasoned salt and seasoning. Grill about 1 minute per side, or until no longer pink inside. Transfer the cutlets to a platter and top with the salsa.

Makes 4 servings

Per serving: 134 calories, 28 g protein, 2 g carbohydrates, 2 g fat (trace saturated), 45 mg cholesterol, 0 g fiber, 155 mg sodium

DATE:

CALORIE GOAL:

WHAT I ATE:

	Calories	Carbohydrate (45%)	Protein (30%)	Fat (25%)
BREAKFAST				
LUNCH				
DINNER				
SNACK 1				
SNACK 2				

TOTAL CALORIES:	+/- GOAL CALORIES:
GLASSES OF WATER	○ ○ ○ ○ ○ ○ ○ ○

WHAT I DID:

	Duration
EXERCISE	

DATE:

CALORIE GOAL:

WHAT I ATE:

	Calories	Carbohydrate (45%)	Protein (30%)	Fat (25%)
BREAKFAST				
LUNCH				
DINNER				
SNACK 1				
SNACK 2				

TOTAL CALORIES:	**+/- GOAL CALORIES:**

GLASSES OF WATER ○ ○ ○ ○ ○ ○ ○ ○

WHAT I DID:

	Duration
EXERCISE	

DATE:

CALORIE GOAL:

WHAT I ATE:

	Calories	Carbohydrate (45%)	Protein (30%)	Fat (25%)
BREAKFAST				
LUNCH				
DINNER				
SNACK 1				
SNACK 2				

TOTAL CALORIES:	+/- GOAL CALORIES:

GLASSES OF WATER ○ ○ ○ ○ ○ ○ ○ ○

WHAT I DID:

	Duration
EXERCISE	

DATE: _____ .   CALORIE GOAL: _____

WHAT I ATE:

	Calories	Carbohydrate (45%)	Protein (30%)	Fat (25%)
BREAKFAST				
LUNCH				
DINNER				
SNACK 1				
SNACK 2				

TOTAL CALORIES:	+/- GOAL CALORIES:
GLASSES OF WATER	○ ○ ○ ○ ○ ○ ○ ○

WHAT I DID:

	Duration
EXERCISE	

DATE:

CALORIE GOAL:

WHAT I ATE:

	Calories	Carbohydrate (45%)	Protein (30%)	Fat (25%)
BREAKFAST				
LUNCH				
DINNER				
SNACK 1				
SNACK 2				

TOTAL CALORIES: **+/- GOAL CALORIES:**

GLASSES OF WATER ○ ○ ○ ○ ○ ○ ○ ○

WHAT I DID:

	Duration
EXERCISE	

PIZZA BURGERS

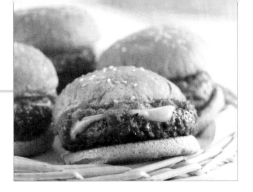

Find a brand of low-fat cheese that you like and stick with it. Using good-quality cheese will ensure that these burgers taste like the real thing.

1	pound 96% lean ground beef
1	teaspoon dried oregano
½	teaspoon garlic powder
½	to 1 teaspoon crushed red pepper flakes, or to taste
¼	teaspoon salt
3	ounces low-fat mozzarella cheese, thinly sliced
½	cup low-fat, reduced-sodium, low-sugar marinara sauce
4	whole grain or whole wheat hamburger buns, split

Preheat a grill to high heat.

In a large bowl, mix the beef, oregano, garlic powder, red pepper flakes, and salt until well combined. Divide the mixture into 4 equal portions and shape into balls, packing them tightly. Press each into a patty about ½" larger than the diameter of the buns.

Grill the burgers for about 2 minutes per side for medium rare, or until desired doneness. (Do not smash the burgers with a spatula.) About 1 minute before they're done, divide the cheese slices among the tops and allow the cheese to melt.

Meanwhile, spoon the sauce into a medium microwaveable bowl. Microwave on low until hot, 30 to 60 seconds. Place the bun halves, cut sides down, on an upper grill rack or away from direct flame for about 20 seconds, or until toasted.

Place each bun bottom on a plate, toasted side up. Place the patties, cheese side up, on top of the bun bottoms. Spread 2 tablespoons sauce on each bun top and place on the patties.

Makes 4 servings

Per serving: 304 calories, 32 g protein, 27 g carbohydrates, 9 g fat (3 g saturated), 68 mg cholesterol, 5 g fiber, 605 mg sodium

DATE:

CALORIE GOAL:

WHAT I ATE:

	Calories	Carbohydrate (45%)	Protein (30%)	Fat (25%)
BREAKFAST				
LUNCH				
DINNER				
SNACK 1				
SNACK 2				

TOTAL CALORIES:	+/- GOAL CALORIES:

GLASSES OF WATER ○ ○ ○ ○ ○ ○ ○ ○

WHAT I DID:

	Duration
EXERCISE	

DATE:

CALORIE GOAL:

WHAT I ATE:

	Calories	Carbohydrate (45%)	Protein (30%)	Fat (25%)
BREAKFAST				
LUNCH				
DINNER				
SNACK 1				
SNACK 2				

TOTAL CALORIES: **+/- GOAL CALORIES:**

GLASSES OF WATER ○ ○ ○ ○ ○ ○ ○ ○

WHAT I DID:

	Duration
EXERCISE	

DATE: | CALORIE GOAL:

WHAT I ATE:

		Calories	Carbohydrate (45%)	Protein (30%)	Fat (25%)
BREAKFAST					
LUNCH					
DINNER					
SNACK 1					
SNACK 2					

TOTAL CALORIES:	+/- GOAL CALORIES:

GLASSES OF WATER ○ ○ ○ ○ ○ ○ ○ ○

WHAT I DID:

		Duration
EXERCISE		

DATE: | CALORIE GOAL:

WHAT I ATE:

	Calories	Carbohydrate (45%)	Protein (30%)	Fat (25%)
BREAKFAST				
LUNCH				
DINNER				
SNACK 1				
SNACK 2				

TOTAL CALORIES:	+/- GOAL CALORIES:
GLASSES OF WATER	○ ○ ○ ○ ○ ○ ○ ○

WHAT I DID:

	Duration
EXERCISE	

DATE:

CALORIE GOAL:

WHAT I ATE:

		Calories	Carbohydrate (45%)	Protein (30%)	Fat (25%)
BREAKFAST					
LUNCH					
DINNER					
SNACK 1					
SNACK 2					

TOTAL CALORIES: **+/- GOAL CALORIES:**

GLASSES OF WATER ○ ○ ○ ○ ○ ○ ○ ○

WHAT I DID:

		Duration
EXERCISE		

WHITE CHICKEN CHILI

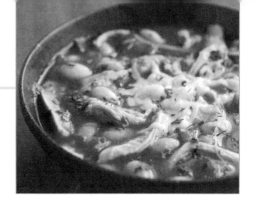

Season 7 contestant Kristin Steede is the brain behind this recipe. You can substitute turkey breast or lean pork loin for the chicken and swap in your favorite beans for endless variations. This recipe is quick and easy, and the chili keeps well in the freezer.

1	pound boneless, skinless chicken breasts or turkey breast, or 1 pound lean pork tenderloin
4½	cups cooked great Northern beans
2	cups fat-free, low-sodium chicken broth
2	cups thick and chunky salsa
1	cup reduced-fat mozzarella cheese
	Chopped cilantro (optional)

Cook and shred the chicken or turkey breast or cook and dice the tenderloin; set aside. In a large saucepan, mix together the beans, broth, and salsa. Heat through and add extra broth, if desired. Stir in the meat and cheese and top with cilantro, if desired. Serve hot.

Makes about 8 (1-cup) servings

Per serving: 230 calories, 26 g protein, 24 g carbohydrates, 4 g fat (2 g saturated), 30 mg cholesterol, 8 g fiber, 230 mg sodium

DATE: _____

CALORIE GOAL: _____

WHAT I ATE:

		Calories	Carbohydrate (45%)	Protein (30%)	Fat (25%)
BREAKFAST					
LUNCH					
DINNER					
SNACK 1					
SNACK 2					

TOTAL CALORIES: _____ **+/- GOAL CALORIES:** _____

GLASSES OF WATER ○ ○ ○ ○ ○ ○ ○ ○

WHAT I DID:

		Duration
EXERCISE		

DATE:

CALORIE GOAL:

WHAT I ATE:

	Calories	Carbohydrate (45%)	Protein (30%)	Fat (25%)
BREAKFAST				
LUNCH				
DINNER				
SNACK 1				
SNACK 2				

TOTAL CALORIES:	+/- GOAL CALORIES:
GLASSES OF WATER	○ ○ ○ ○ ○ ○ ○ ○

WHAT I DID:

	Duration
EXERCISE	

DATE:

CALORIE GOAL:

WHAT I ATE:

		Calories	Carbohydrate (45%)	Protein (30%)	Fat (25%)
BREAKFAST					
LUNCH					
DINNER					
SNACK 1					
SNACK 2					

TOTAL CALORIES: **+/- GOAL CALORIES:**

GLASSES OF WATER ○ ○ ○ ○ ○ ○ ○ ○

WHAT I DID:

	Duration
EXERCISE	

DATE:

CALORIE GOAL:

WHAT I ATE:

	Calories	Carbohydrate (45%)	Protein (30%)	Fat (25%)
BREAKFAST				
LUNCH				
DINNER				
SNACK 1				
SNACK 2				

TOTAL CALORIES:	+/- GOAL CALORIES:

GLASSES OF WATER	○ ○ ○ ○ ○ ○ ○ ○

WHAT I DID:

	Duration
EXERCISE	

DATE:

CALORIE GOAL:

WHAT I ATE:

	Calories	Carbohydrate (45%)	Protein (30%)	Fat (25%)
BREAKFAST				
LUNCH				
DINNER				
SNACK 1				
SNACK 2				

TOTAL CALORIES: **+/- GOAL CALORIES:**

GLASSES OF WATER   ○ ○ ○ ○ ○ ○ ○ ○

WHAT I DID:

	Duration
EXERCISE	

CHEESY BAKED SWEET POTATO

Sweet potatoes contain dietary fiber and protein and are a source of vitamins A and C, iron, and calcium. This delicious version of a classic baked potato makes a light yet satisfying vegetarian meal when paired with a side salad. If you have trouble finding a sweet potato that's exactly 6 ounces, you can follow the directions below and make two servings using two wedges of cheese and one 12-ounce potato. (The larger potato will take a bit longer to cook in the microwave.)

1   (6-ounce) sweet potato, scrubbed

1   wedge (¾ ounce) Laughing Cow Light Garlic and Herb cheese

With a fork, poke the potato 5 times on each side. Place in a microwaveable bowl or dish. Cover the bowl loosely with a paper towel and microwave on high for 5 minutes. Carefully flip the potato (it will be very hot) and microwave for 3 to 5 minutes more, or until it is tender throughout.

Cut an opening in the center of the potato, leaving 1" uncut at each end but penetrating deeply enough to open the potato completely without cutting it in half. Spread the cheese evenly in the center and mash it into the potato slightly with a fork to melt.

Makes 1 serving

Per serving: 166 calories, 5 g protein, 31 g carbohydrates, 2 g fat (1 g saturated), 10 mg cholesterol, 5 g fiber, 352 mg sodium

Recipe excerpted from *The Biggest Loser: Family Cookbook.*

For more ways to live *The Biggest Loser* lifestyle, go to biggestloser.com.

DATE:

CALORIE GOAL:

WHAT I ATE:

	Calories	Carbohydrate (45%)	Protein (30%)	Fat (25%)
BREAKFAST				
LUNCH				
DINNER				
SNACK 1				
SNACK 2				

TOTAL CALORIES: **+/- GOAL CALORIES:**

GLASSES OF WATER ○ ○ ○ ○ ○ ○ ○ ○

WHAT I DID:

	Duration
EXERCISE	

DATE:

CALORIE GOAL:

WHAT I ATE:

	Calories	Carbohydrate (45%)	Protein (30%)	Fat (25%)
BREAKFAST				
LUNCH				
DINNER				
SNACK 1				
SNACK 2				

TOTAL CALORIES: **+/- GOAL CALORIES:**

GLASSES OF WATER ○ ○ ○ ○ ○ ○ ○ ○

WHAT I DID:

	Duration
EXERCISE	

DATE: _____ CALORIE GOAL: _____

WHAT I ATE:

	Calories	Carbohydrate (45%)	Protein (30%)	Fat (25%)
BREAKFAST				
LUNCH				
DINNER				
SNACK 1				
SNACK 2				

TOTAL CALORIES:	+/- GOAL CALORIES:

GLASSES OF WATER ○ ○ ○ ○ ○ ○ ○ ○

WHAT I DID:

	Duration
EXERCISE	

DATE:

CALORIE GOAL:

WHAT I ATE:

	Calories	Carbohydrate (45%)	Protein (30%)	Fat (25%)
BREAKFAST				
LUNCH				
DINNER				
SNACK 1				
SNACK 2				

TOTAL CALORIES: **+/- GOAL CALORIES:**

GLASSES OF WATER ○ ○ ○ ○ ○ ○ ○ ○

WHAT I DID:

	Duration
EXERCISE	

DATE:

CALORIE GOAL:

WHAT I ATE:

	Calories	Carbohydrate (45%)	Protein (30%)	Fat (25%)
BREAKFAST				
LUNCH				
DINNER				
SNACK 1				
SNACK 2				

TOTAL CALORIES: **+/- GOAL CALORIES:**

GLASSES OF WATER   ○ ○ ○ ○ ○ ○ ○ ○

WHAT I DID:

	Duration
EXERCISE	

ROSEMARY-ROASTED ROOT VEGETABLES

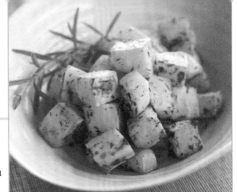

The secret to perfect roasting is a hot oven and a large enough pan to eliminate crowding. This ensures a crispy exterior and even browning. You can change the proportions of the vegetables if you like; just be sure they're cut the same size for uniform baking. Butternut squash or sweet potatoes work well, too.

16	ounces any combination of parsnips, rutabagas, and turnips, peeled and cut in 1" pieces
2	teaspoons olive oil
1	teaspoon chopped fresh rosemary
1	teaspoon chopped fresh thyme
½	teaspoon mustard powder
¼	teaspoon salt
¼	teaspoon ground black pepper

Preheat the oven to 400°F. Place the parsnips, rutabagas, and turnips on a 15" × 10" baking sheet. Drizzle with the oil and sprinkle with the rosemary, thyme, mustard, and salt. Toss well and distribute evenly over the pan. Roast, stirring or shaking the vegetables every 15 minutes, until they're tender and evenly browned, or about 45 minutes. Sprinkle with black pepper; taste and adjust the seasonings. Serve hot or at room temperature.

Makes 4 servings

Per serving: 70 calories, 1 g protein, 13 g carbohydrates, 2 g fat (0 g saturated), 0 mg cholesterol, 3 g fiber, 180 mg sodium

DATE:

CALORIE GOAL:

WHAT I ATE:

	Calories	Carbohydrate (45%)	Protein (30%)	Fat (25%)
BREAKFAST				
LUNCH				
DINNER				
SNACK 1				
SNACK 2				

TOTAL CALORIES: **+/- GOAL CALORIES:**

GLASSES OF WATER ○ ○ ○ ○ ○ ○ ○ ○

WHAT I DID:

	Duration
EXERCISE	

DATE:

CALORIE GOAL:

WHAT I ATE:

	Calories	Carbohydrate (45%)	Protein (30%)	Fat (25%)
BREAKFAST				
LUNCH				
DINNER				
SNACK 1				
SNACK 2				

TOTAL CALORIES:	+/- GOAL CALORIES:

GLASSES OF WATER	○ ○ ○ ○ ○ ○ ○ ○

WHAT I DID:

	Duration
EXERCISE	

DATE: _____

CALORIE GOAL: _____

WHAT I ATE:

	Calories	Carbohydrate (45%)	Protein (30%)	Fat (25%)
BREAKFAST				
LUNCH				
DINNER				
SNACK 1				
SNACK 2				

TOTAL CALORIES: _____ **+/- GOAL CALORIES:** _____

GLASSES OF WATER ○ ○ ○ ○ ○ ○ ○ ○

WHAT I DID:

	Duration
EXERCISE	

DATE:

CALORIE GOAL:

WHAT I ATE:

	Calories	Carbohydrate (45%)	Protein (30%)	Fat (25%)
BREAKFAST				
LUNCH				
DINNER				
SNACK 1				
SNACK 2				

TOTAL CALORIES: +/- GOAL CALORIES:

GLASSES OF WATER ○ ○ ○ ○ ○ ○ ○ ○

WHAT I DID:

	Duration
EXERCISE	

DATE: _____

CALORIE GOAL: _____

WHAT I ATE:

	Calories	Carbohydrate (45%)	Protein (30%)	Fat (25%)
BREAKFAST				
LUNCH				
DINNER				
SNACK 1				
SNACK 2				

TOTAL CALORIES: _____ **+/- GOAL CALORIES:** _____

GLASSES OF WATER ○ ○ ○ ○ ○ ○ ○ ○

WHAT I DID:

	Duration
EXERCISE	

BRUSSELS SPROUTS WITH TOASTED HAZELNUTS

At only 20 calories, ½ cup of brussels sprouts packs a big nutrient bang, with 3 grams of fiber and 60 percent of the daily requirement for vitamin C.

- 1 pound fresh (or thawed frozen) brussels sprouts
- 1 tablespoon extra-virgin olive oil
- 3 tablespoons chopped shallots
- Salt and pepper to taste

- ⅛ teaspoon ground nutmeg
- 1 teaspoon agave nectar, honey, or maple syrup
- 1 tablespoon chopped hazelnuts, toasted
- 2 teaspoons grated orange peel

Bring 2 quarts of salted water to a boil.

Remove the outer leaves from the sprouts and trim the ends of the bases. Quarter the sprouts vertically, leaving the cores intact.

Add the brussels sprouts to the boiling water and cook for about 3 minutes, or until fork-tender. Drain and immediately transfer to enough cold water to cover them. The brussels sprouts can be prepared in advance up to this point and refrigerated.

Heat the oil in a skillet over medium-high heat. Cook the shallots in the oil for about 2 minutes, or just until softened. Add the brussels sprouts and cook for about 2 minutes, or until they are heated through. (It will take slightly longer if the sprouts were cooked and refrigerated in advance.) Season with salt, pepper, and nutmeg. Drizzle the agave nectar over the brussels sprouts and stir well. Garnish with the toasted nuts and orange peel.

Makes 4 (¾-cup) servings

Per serving: 100 calories, 4 g protein, 12 g carbohydrates, 5 g fat (less than 1 g saturated), 0 mg cholesterol, 5 g fiber, 310 mg sodium

DATE: _____

CALORIE GOAL: _____

WHAT I ATE:

	Calories	Carbohydrate (45%)	Protein (30%)	Fat (25%)
BREAKFAST				
LUNCH				
DINNER				
SNACK 1				
SNACK 2				

TOTAL CALORIES: _____ +/- GOAL CALORIES: _____

GLASSES OF WATER ○ ○ ○ ○ ○ ○ ○ ○

WHAT I DID:

	Duration
EXERCISE	

DATE:

CALORIE GOAL:

WHAT I ATE:

	Calories	Carbohydrate (45%)	Protein (30%)	Fat (25%)
BREAKFAST				
LUNCH				
DINNER				
SNACK 1				
SNACK 2				

TOTAL CALORIES: **+/- GOAL CALORIES:**

GLASSES OF WATER   ◯ ◯ ◯ ◯ ◯ ◯ ◯ ◯

WHAT I DID:

	Duration
EXERCISE	

DATE: _____

CALORIE GOAL: _____

WHAT I ATE:

		Calories	Carbohydrate (45%)	Protein (30%)	Fat (25%)
BREAKFAST					
LUNCH					
DINNER					
SNACK 1					
SNACK 2					

TOTAL CALORIES: _____ **+/- GOAL CALORIES:** _____

GLASSES OF WATER ○ ○ ○ ○ ○ ○ ○ ○

WHAT I DID:

		Duration
EXERCISE		

DATE:

CALORIE GOAL:

WHAT I ATE:

	Calories	Carbohydrate (45%)	Protein (30%)	Fat (25%)
BREAKFAST				
LUNCH				
DINNER				
SNACK 1				
SNACK 2				

TOTAL CALORIES:　　　　**+/- GOAL CALORIES:**

GLASSES OF WATER　○　○　○　○　○　○　○　○

WHAT I DID:

	Duration
EXERCISE	

DATE: _____

CALORIE GOAL: _____

WHAT I ATE:

	Calories	Carbohydrate (45%)	Protein (30%)	Fat (25%)
BREAKFAST				
LUNCH				
DINNER				
SNACK 1				
SNACK 2				

TOTAL CALORIES: _____ **+/- GOAL CALORIES:** _____

GLASSES OF WATER ○ ○ ○ ○ ○ ○ ○ ○

WHAT I DID:

	Duration
EXERCISE	

FROSTY PUMPKIN SMOOTHIE

The rich flavors of this smoothie are truly reminiscent of pumpkin pie—in a glass! It will satisfy your sweet tooth while delivering a healthy dose of calcium and vitamin A.

½   cup pumpkin puree, fresh or canned

½   cup fat-free milk

2   tablespoons agave nectar

½   teaspoon vanilla extract

¼   teaspoon ground cinnamon

⅛   teaspoon ground ginger

⅛   teaspoon ground cloves

5   ice cubes

½   cup fat-free Greek-style plain yogurt + extra for garnish

Pinch of ground nutmeg

Combine the pumpkin, milk, nectar, vanilla extract, cinnamon, ginger, cloves, ice, and ½ cup yogurt in a blender and blend until smooth. Pour the smoothie into a chilled glass and garnish with a dollop of yogurt and a sprinkle of nutmeg.

Makes 2 servings (about 2 cups)

Per serving: 130 calories, 8 g protein, 26 g carbohydrates, 0 g fat (0 g saturated), 0 mg cholesterol, 2 g fiber, 45 mg sodium

DATE:

CALORIE GOAL:

WHAT I ATE:

	Calories	Carbohydrate (45%)	Protein (30%)	Fat (25%)
BREAKFAST				
LUNCH				
DINNER				
SNACK 1				
SNACK 2				

TOTAL CALORIES: **+/- GOAL CALORIES:**

GLASSES OF WATER ○ ○ ○ ○ ○ ○ ○ ○

WHAT I DID:

	Duration
EXERCISE	

DATE:

CALORIE GOAL:

WHAT I ATE:

	Calories	Carbohydrate (45%)	Protein (30%)	Fat (25%)
BREAKFAST				
LUNCH				
DINNER				
SNACK 1				
SNACK 2				

TOTAL CALORIES: **+/- GOAL CALORIES:**

GLASSES OF WATER   ◯ ◯ ◯ ◯ ◯ ◯ ◯ ◯

WHAT I DID:

	Duration
EXERCISE	

DATE:

CALORIE GOAL:

WHAT I ATE:

		Calories	Carbohydrate (45%)	Protein (30%)	Fat (25%)
BREAKFAST					
LUNCH					
DINNER					
SNACK 1					
SNACK 2					

TOTAL CALORIES:	+/- GOAL CALORIES:
GLASSES OF WATER	○ ○ ○ ○ ○ ○ ○ ○

WHAT I DID:

	Duration
EXERCISE	

DATE:

WHAT I ATE:

	Calories	Carbohydrate (45%)	Protein (30%)	Fat (25%)
BREAKFAST				
LUNCH				
DINNER				
SNACK 1				
SNACK 2				

TOTAL CALORIES: **+/- GOAL CALORIES:**

GLASSES OF WATER   ◯ ◯ ◯ ◯ ◯ ◯ ◯ ◯

WHAT I DID:

	Duration
EXERCISE	

DATE:

WHAT I ATE:

		Calories	Carbohydrate (45%)	Protein (30%)	Fat (25%)
BREAKFAST					
LUNCH					
DINNER					
SNACK 1					
SNACK 2					

TOTAL CALORIES: **+/- GOAL CALORIES:**

GLASSES OF WATER   ○ ○ ○ ○ ○ ○ ○ ○

WHAT I DID:

		Duration
EXERCISE		

JERRY AND ESTELLA'S CHERRY CRUNCH

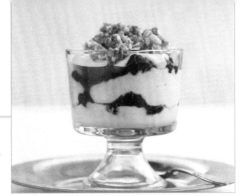

This recipe is a routine Simple Swap that Jerry and Estella Hayes of Season 7 created to replace their old after-dinner ice cream routine. Simple, crunchy, and sweet, it's their favorite choice for those nights when they have enough calories left in their daily budget for a sweet indulgence.

- 1   **cup frozen or fresh sweet cherries, pitted**
- ¾   **cup fat-free Greek-style yogurt**
- 2   **teaspoons (2 packets) Truvia Natural Sweetener or other natural sweetener**
- ½   **cup Kashi GoLean Crunch cereal**

Heat the frozen cherries in the microwave in a microwave-safe container for about 30 seconds. Combine the yogurt and sweetener. In a parfait glass, layer the yogurt and cherries and top with the cereal. Serve immediately.

Makes 2 (¾-cup) servings

Per serving: 130 calories, 11 g protein, 23 g carbohydrates, 1 g fat (0 g saturated), 0 mg cholesterol, 4 g fiber, 80 mg sodium

Recipe excerpted from *The Biggest Loser: Simple Swaps.*

For more ways to live *The Biggest Loser* lifestyle, go to biggestloser.com.

DATE: |||||| CALORIE GOAL:

WHAT I ATE:

		Calories	Carbohydrate (45%)	Protein (30%)	Fat (25%)
BREAKFAST					
LUNCH					
DINNER					
SNACK 1					
SNACK 2					

TOTAL CALORIES:	+/- GOAL CALORIES:

GLASSES OF WATER ○ ○ ○ ○ ○ ○ ○ ○

WHAT I DID:

		Duration
EXERCISE		

DATE:

CALORIE GOAL:

WHAT I ATE:

	Calories	Carbohydrate (45%)	Protein (30%)	Fat (25%)
BREAKFAST				
LUNCH				
DINNER				
SNACK 1				
SNACK 2				

TOTAL CALORIES: **+/- GOAL CALORIES:**

GLASSES OF WATER ○ ○ ○ ○ ○ ○ ○ ○

WHAT I DID:

	Duration
EXERCISE	

DATE:

CALORIE GOAL:

WHAT I ATE:

	Calories	Carbohydrate (45%)	Protein (30%)	Fat (25%)
BREAKFAST				
LUNCH				
DINNER				
SNACK 1				
SNACK 2				

TOTAL CALORIES:	**+/- GOAL CALORIES:**

GLASSES OF WATER ○ ○ ○ ○ ○ ○ ○ ○

WHAT I DID:

	Duration
EXERCISE	

DATE:

CALORIE GOAL:

WHAT I ATE:

	Calories	Carbohydrate (45%)	Protein (30%)	Fat (25%)
BREAKFAST				
LUNCH				
DINNER				
SNACK 1				
SNACK 2				

TOTAL CALORIES: +/- GOAL CALORIES:

GLASSES OF WATER   ○ ○ ○ ○ ○ ○ ○ ○

WHAT I DID:

	Duration
EXERCISE	

DATE:

CALORIE GOAL:

WHAT I ATE:

		Calories	Carbohydrate (45%)	Protein (30%)	Fat (25%)
BREAKFAST					
LUNCH					
DINNER					
SNACK 1					
SNACK 2					

TOTAL CALORIES: **+/- GOAL CALORIES:**

GLASSES OF WATER ○ ○ ○ ○ ○ ○ ○ ○

WHAT I DID:

		Duration
EXERCISE		

MAPLE RICOTTA CHEESECAKES WITH BERRIES AND TOASTED PECANS

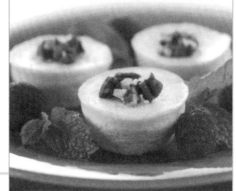

Using fat-free ricotta cheese and nonfat yogurt rather than regular cream cheese and sour cream gives this recipe far less fat than you'll find in a traditional cheesecake.

2 cups fat-free ricotta cheese

1 cup (8 ounces) light cream cheese

½ cup fat-free Greek-style plain yogurt

½ cup maple syrup

1 large whole egg

3 large egg whites

2 teaspoons vanilla extract

1½ cups fresh berries

2 tablespoons chopped toasted pecans

Fresh mint sprigs

Preheat the oven to 325°F. Lightly coat 3 mini-muffin pans with cooking spray.

Add the ricotta, cream cheese, yogurt, syrup, egg, egg whites, and vanilla extract to a blender or food processor. Blend or process just until smooth. Divide the batter among the prepared pans. The batter will come to the top of the cups.

Bake for 20 minutes. Cool completely, then chill. It's normal for the cheesecakes to fall.

To serve, place 3 cakes on each plate. Garnish with berries, nuts, and mint.

Makes 12 (3-cheesecake) servings

Per serving: 140 calories, 8 g protein, 16 g carbohydrates, 5 g fat (3 g saturated), 35 mg cholesterol, 3 g fiber, 125 mg sodium

DATE: _____

CALORIE GOAL: _____

WHAT I ATE:

		Calories	Carbohydrate (45%)	Protein (30%)	Fat (25%)
BREAKFAST					
LUNCH					
DINNER					
SNACK 1					
SNACK 2					

TOTAL CALORIES: _____ **+/- GOAL CALORIES:** _____

GLASSES OF WATER ○ ○ ○ ○ ○ ○ ○ ○

WHAT I DID:

	Duration
EXERCISE	

DATE: _____

WHAT I ATE:

	Calories	Carbohydrate (45%)	Protein (30%)	Fat (25%)
BREAKFAST				
LUNCH				
DINNER				
SNACK 1				
SNACK 2				

TOTAL CALORIES: _____ **+/- GOAL CALORIES:** _____

GLASSES OF WATER   ○ ○ ○ ○ ○ ○ ○ ○

WHAT I DID:

	Duration
EXERCISE	

DATE:

CALORIE GOAL:

WHAT I ATE:

	Calories	Carbohydrate (45%)	Protein (30%)	Fat (25%)
BREAKFAST				
LUNCH				
DINNER				
SNACK 1				
SNACK 2				

TOTAL CALORIES: **+/- GOAL CALORIES:**

GLASSES OF WATER   ◯ ◯ ◯ ◯ ◯ ◯ ◯ ◯

WHAT I DID:

	Duration
EXERCISE	

DATE: _____

CALORIE GOAL: _____

WHAT I ATE:

	Calories	Carbohydrate (45%)	Protein (30%)	Fat (25%)
BREAKFAST				
LUNCH				
DINNER				
SNACK 1				
SNACK 2				

TOTAL CALORIES: _____ **+/- GOAL CALORIES:** _____

GLASSES OF WATER ○ ○ ○ ○ ○ ○ ○ ○

WHAT I DID:

	Duration
EXERCISE	

DATE:

CALORIE GOAL:

WHAT I ATE:

	Calories	Carbohydrate (45%)	Protein (30%)	Fat (25%)
BREAKFAST				
LUNCH				
DINNER				
SNACK 1				
SNACK 2				

TOTAL CALORIES: +/- GOAL CALORIES:

GLASSES OF WATER   ○ ○ ○ ○ ○ ○ ○ ○

WHAT I DID:

EXERCISE	Duration

VANILLA POACHED PEARS

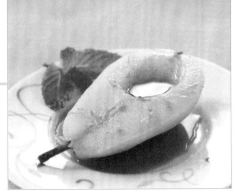

The Biggest Losers are encouraged to eat fruit for dessert. This sweet, delicious pear dish is fancy enough to serve to guests yet basic enough to make on a weeknight.

1 cup water

1 cup unsweetened apple juice

¼ cup agave nectar or dark honey

2 tablespoons orange juice

1 teaspoon vanilla extract

½ teaspoon ground cinnamon

Pinch of cloves

2 tablespoons grated orange peel

4 firm, ripe pears

2 tablespoons lemon juice

Fresh mint leaves

In a 3-quart saucepan over medium heat, combine the water, apple juice, nectar, orange juice, vanilla extract, cinnamon, cloves, and 1 tablespoon of the orange peel. Bring to a boil.

While the poaching liquid is coming to a boil, peel, halve, and core the pears and immediately coat them in lemon juice.

Reduce the poaching liquid to a simmer, add the pears, cover, and simmer for 2 minutes. Remove the pears from the heat and allow them to cool in the juices. Remove the pears from the pan. Heat the juice to reduce it by half. Strain it and pour it over the pears. Garnish with the remaining orange peel and fresh mint, and enjoy hot or cold.

Makes 8 servings

Per serving: 110 calories, 1 g protein, 23 g carbohydrates, less than 1 g fat (0 g saturated), 0 mg cholesterol, 2 g fiber, 0 mg sodium

DATE: _____

CALORIE GOAL: _____

WHAT I ATE:

	Calories	Carbohydrate (45%)	Protein (30%)	Fat (25%)
BREAKFAST				
LUNCH				
DINNER				
SNACK 1				
SNACK 2				

TOTAL CALORIES: _____ **+/- GOAL CALORIES:** _____

GLASSES OF WATER ○ ○ ○ ○ ○ ○ ○ ○

WHAT I DID:

	Duration
EXERCISE	

DATE:

CALORIE GOAL:

WHAT I ATE:

	Calories	Carbohydrate (45%)	Protein (30%)	Fat (25%)
BREAKFAST				
LUNCH				
DINNER				
SNACK 1				
SNACK 2				

TOTAL CALORIES: **+/- GOAL CALORIES:**

GLASSES OF WATER ○ ○ ○ ○ ○ ○ ○ ○

WHAT I DID:

	Duration
EXERCISE	

DATE: _____

CALORIE GOAL: _____

WHAT I ATE:

	Calories	Carbohydrate (45%)	Protein (30%)	Fat (25%)
BREAKFAST				
LUNCH				
DINNER				
SNACK 1				
SNACK 2				

TOTAL CALORIES: _____ **+/- GOAL CALORIES:** _____

GLASSES OF WATER ○ ○ ○ ○ ○ ○ ○ ○

WHAT I DID:

	Duration
EXERCISE	

DATE:

CALORIE GOAL:

WHAT I ATE:

		Calories	Carbohydrate (45%)	Protein (30%)	Fat (25%)
BREAKFAST					
LUNCH					
DINNER					
SNACK 1					
SNACK 2					

TOTAL CALORIES: **+/- GOAL CALORIES:**

GLASSES OF WATER ○ ○ ○ ○ ○ ○ ○ ○

WHAT I DID:

	Duration
EXERCISE	

DATE:

CALORIE GOAL:

WHAT I ATE:

	Calories	Carbohydrate (45%)	Protein (30%)	Fat (25%)
BREAKFAST				
LUNCH				
DINNER				
SNACK 1				
SNACK 2				

TOTAL CALORIES: **+/- GOAL CALORIES:**

GLASSES OF WATER   ○ ○ ○ ○ ○ ○ ○ ○

WHAT I DID:

	Duration
EXERCISE	

EASY RASPBERRY SORBET

"I can't cook" is no excuse when making dessert is this simple. Try substituting different berries or fruits, such as peaches or mangoes, for other limitless flavor possibilities.

- **2**   **cups frozen raspberries or other frozen fruit**
- **3**   **tablespoons apple juice or orange juice**
- **½**   **teaspoon cinnamon or pure vanilla extract (optional)**
       Fresh mint leaves

Place the frozen fruit, the juice, and the cinnamon or vanilla extract (if desired) in a blender or food processor. Blend or process until smooth, scraping down the sides of the container as necessary. Add extra juice if needed. The sorbet is best if served immediately, although it can be frozen. Garnish with fresh mint.

Makes 4 servings

Per serving: 35 calories, 1 g protein, 9 g carbohydrates (3 g sugars), 0 g fat (0 g saturated), 0 mg cholesterol, 4 g fiber, 1 mg sodium

DATE:

CALORIE GOAL:

WHAT I ATE:

		Calories	Carbohydrate (45%)	Protein (30%)	Fat (25%)
BREAKFAST					
LUNCH					
DINNER					
SNACK 1					
SNACK 2					

TOTAL CALORIES: **+/- GOAL CALORIES:**

GLASSES OF WATER ○ ○ ○ ○ ○ ○ ○ ○

WHAT I DID:

	Duration
EXERCISE	

DATE:

CALORIE GOAL:

WHAT I ATE:

	Calories	Carbohydrate (45%)	Protein (30%)	Fat (25%)
BREAKFAST				
LUNCH				
DINNER				
SNACK 1				
SNACK 2				

TOTAL CALORIES: **+/- GOAL CALORIES:**

GLASSES OF WATER   ○ ○ ○ ○ ○ ○ ○ ○

WHAT I DID:

	Duration
EXERCISE	

DATE:

CALORIE GOAL:

WHAT I ATE:

	Calories	Carbohydrate (45%)	Protein (30%)	Fat (25%)
BREAKFAST				
LUNCH				
DINNER				
SNACK 1				
SNACK 2				

TOTAL CALORIES: **+/- GOAL CALORIES:**

GLASSES OF WATER ○ ○ ○ ○ ○ ○ ○ ○

WHAT I DID:

	Duration
EXERCISE	

DATE: _____

WHAT I ATE:

	Calories	Carbohydrate (45%)	Protein (30%)	Fat (25%)
BREAKFAST				
LUNCH				
DINNER				
SNACK 1				
SNACK 2				

TOTAL CALORIES:		**+/- GOAL CALORIES:**	
GLASSES OF WATER	○ ○ ○ ○ ○ ○ ○ ○		

WHAT I DID:

	Duration
EXERCISE	

DATE: _____

CALORIE GOAL: _____

WHAT I ATE:

		Calories	Carbohydrate (45%)	Protein (30%)	Fat (25%)
BREAKFAST					
LUNCH					
DINNER					
SNACK 1					
SNACK 2					

TOTAL CALORIES:	+/- GOAL CALORIES:

GLASSES OF WATER ○ ○ ○ ○ ○ ○ ○ ○

WHAT I DID:

		Duration
EXERCISE		

MINI APPLE GINGERBREAD CUPCAKES

These irresistible little cakes are spicy but not too sweet. For sweeter flavor, you can add an additional tablespoon of your favorite natural sweetener to the batter.

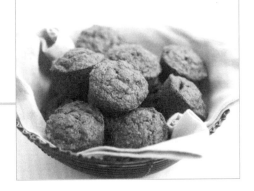

2 cups stone-ground whole wheat flour

1 teaspoon baking soda

¼ teaspoon salt

2 teaspoons ground ginger

1 teaspoon ground cinnamon

¼ teaspoon ground cloves

¼ teaspoon ground nutmeg

⅔ cup low-fat buttermilk

½ cup molasses

⅓ cup canola oil

1 large egg

1 large egg white

1 teaspoon vanilla extract

1 cup finely chopped apple (sweet variety such as Fuji or Delicious, not Granny Smith)

Preheat the oven to 350°F. Lightly coat 2½ mini-muffin pans with cooking spray.

In a medium mixing bowl, combine the dry ingredients. Set aside.

In another bowl, whisk together the buttermilk, molasses, oil, egg, egg white, and vanilla extract. Make a well in the dry ingredients and pour in the liquid mixture. Stir in the apple until just combined. Divide the batter among the prepared muffin pans.

Bake on the center rack for about 15 minutes, or until a wooden pick inserted in a cupcake comes out clean. Cool for about 10 minutes before removing from the pans.

Makes 30 (1-mini-cupcake) servings

Per serving: 70 calories, 1 g protein, 10 g carbohydrates, 2 g fat (0 g saturated), 0 mg cholesterol, 1 g fiber, 90 mg sodium

APPENDIX

CONVERSION TABLE FOR MEASURING PORTION SIZES

Teaspoons	Tablespoons	Cups	Pints, quarts, gallons	Fluid ounces	Milliliters
¼ teaspoon					1 milliliter
½ teaspoon					2 milliliters
1 teaspoon	⅓ tablespoon				5 milliliters
3 teaspoons	1 tablespoon	¹⁄₁₆ cup		½ ounce	15 milliliters
6 teaspoons	2 tablespoons	⅛ cup		1 ounce	30 milliliters
12 teaspoons	4 tablespoons	¼ cup		2 ounces	60 milliliters
16 teaspoons	5⅓ tablespoons	⅓ cup		2½ ounces	75 milliliters
24 teaspoons	8 tablespoons	½ cup		4 ounces	125 milliliters
32 teaspoons	10⅔ tablespoons	⅔ cup		5 ounces	150 milliliters
36 teaspoons	12 tablespoons	¾ cup		6 ounces	175 milliliters
48 teaspoons	16 tablespoons	1 cup	½ pint	8 ounces	237 milliliters
		2 cups	1 pint	16 ounces	473 milliliters
		3 cups		24 ounces	710 milliliters
		4 cups	1 quart	32 ounces	946 milliliters
		8 cups	½ gallon	64 ounces	
		16 cups	1 gallon	128 ounces	

FIBER CONTENT OF COMMON WHOLE GRAINS

Grain (¼ cup uncooked)	Fiber (grams)
Barley	8
Bulgur	6
Wheat germ	4
Whole wheat couscous	4
Quinoa	3
Wild rice	3
Cream of wheat	2
High-fiber cornmeal	2
Rolled oats	2

CAFFEINE CONTENT OF COMMON BEVERAGES

Beverage or other product	Serving size	Caffeine content (mcg)
Coffee, brewed	8 ounces	137
Black tea, brewed	8 ounces	65
Iced tea, black, instant	8 ounces	47
Espresso	2 ounces	42
Dark chocolate, bittersweet	1 ounce	20
Green tea, brewed	8 ounces	40
Natural unsweetened cocoa powder	1 tablespoon	12
Decaf green tea	8 ounces	5
Decaf coffee, brewed	8 ounces	2
Diet soda	12 ounces	46
Coca-Cola Classic	12 ounces	34

CALORIE COUNTS OF COMMON FOODS

Food Item	Serving Size	Calories	Protein (g)	Carb (g)	Fiber (g)	Sugars (g)	Fat (g)	Sat Fat (g)	Sodium (mg)
Beans and Legumes									
cannellini beans, cooked without salt	½ cup	100	6	17	5	1	1	0	40
chickpeas (garbanzo beans), cooked without salt	½ cup	134	7	22	6	4	2	0	6
edamame, out of shell, cooked with salt	½ cup	100	8	9	4	1	3	1	225
hummus	⅛ cup	56	3	6	1	0	3	0	76
hummus, low-fat	⅛ cup	59	5	6	2	0	2.5	0	111
kidney beans, red, cooked without salt	½ cup	110	8	20	8	0	0	0	4
navy beans, cooked without salt	½ cup	127	7	10	0	0	1	0	0
pinto beans, cooked without salt	½ cup	122	8	22	8	0	1	0	1
refried beans, fat-free	½ cup	130	9	24	7	0	0	0	490

Food Item	Serving Size	Calories	Protein (g)	Carb (g)	Fiber (g)	Sugars (g)	Fat (g)	Sat Fat (g)	Sodium (mg)
Beverages: Alcoholic									
beer, dark	12 fl oz	150	1	13	n/a	n/a	0	0	34
beer, lager	12 fl oz	102	1	6	1	0	0	0	14
beer, light	12 fl oz	110	1	7	0	n/a	0	0	11
wine, red	5 fl oz	125	0	4	0	1	0	0	6
wine, white, medium	5 fl oz	122	0	4	0	1	0	0	7
Beverages: Coffees and Teas									
cappuccino, with fat-free milk	8 fl oz	53	5	7	0	7	0	0	73
coffee, brewed	8 fl oz	2	0	0	0	0	0	0	0
coffee, decaf, brewed	8 fl oz	0	0	0	0	0	0	0	0
coffee, instant	1 Tbsp	7	0	1	0	0	0	0	1
coffee, latte, with fat-free milk	8 fl oz	47	5	7	0	6	0	0	67
espresso	4 fl oz	11	0	2	0	2	0	0	17
tea, herbal	8 fl oz	2	0	0	0	0	0	0	2
Beverages: Juices									
apple juice, unsweetened	4 fl oz	58	0	14	0	14	0	0	4
carrot juice	4 fl oz	47	1	11	1	5	0	0	34

Food Item	Serving Size	Calories	Protein (g)	Carb (g)	Fiber (g)	Sugars (g)	Fat (g)	Sat Fat (g)	Sodium (mg)
Beverages: Juices—*Continued*									
cranberry juice cocktail	4 fl oz	68	0	17	0	15	0	0	3
grapefruit juice, white	4 fl oz	48	1	11	0	11	0	0	1
grape juice drink	4 fl oz	71	0	18	0	18	0	0	11
lemon juice	4 fl oz	30	0	10	0	3	0	0	1
lime juice	4 fl oz	31	1	10	0	2	0	0	2
orange juice	4 fl oz	56	1	13	0	10	0	0	1
pomegranate juice	4 fl oz	70	1	18	0	17	0	0	15
tomato-vegetable juice, low-sodium	4 fl oz	25	1	5	1	4	0	0	70
Beverages: Milk and Nondairy Milk									
cocoa, hot, with fat-free milk	8 fl oz	138	8	27	1	n/a	1	1	146
half-and-half, fat-free	1 fl oz	37	1	1	0	1	0	0	14
milk, fat-free	1 cup	90	9	13	0	12	0	0	130
milk, 1% (low-fat)	1 cup	118	10	14	0	11	3	2	143

Food Item	Serving Size	Calories	Protein (g)	Carb (g)	Fiber (g)	Sugars (g)	Fat (g)	Sat Fat (g)	Sodium (mg)
milk, 1% (low-fat), lactose-reduced	1 cup	103	8	12	0	12	3	2	124
milk, 2% (reduced-fat)	1 cup	122	8	11	0	11	5	3	100
nondairy almond milk, Almond Breeze	1 cup	63	1	8	1	7	3	0	153
rice milk	1 cup	144	3	28	2	n/a	2	0	86
soy milk	1 cup	127	11	12	3	1	5	1	135
soy milk, Silk, vanilla	1 cup	100	6	10	1	7	3.5	0.5	95
Breads and Crackers									
bagel, cinnamon raisin	1 oz	22	3	16	1	2	0	0	91
bagel, plain	1 oz	81	3	16	1	2	0	0	136
bagel, whole grain	1 oz	75	3	16	3	1	0	0	153
bread, Ezekiel 4:9 Sprouted Grain	1 slice (34 g)	80	4	15	3	n/a	1	0	75
bread, pita, whole wheat	½ of 6½" pita (1 oz)	85	3	18	2	0	1	0	170

Food Item	Serving Size	Calories	Protein (g)	Carb (g)	Fiber (g)	Sugars (g)	Fat (g)	Sat Fat (g)	Sodium (mg)
		Breads and Crackers—*Continued*							
bread, pumpernickel	1 slice (1 oz)	65	2	12	2	0	1	0	174
bread, rye	1 slice (1 oz)	82	3	15	2	1	1	0	211
bread, seven-grain	1 slice (1 oz)	65	3	12	2	3	1	0	127
bread, white	1 slice (1 oz)	67	2	13	1	1	1	0	170
bread, white, reduced-calorie	2 slices (2 oz)	95	4	20	4	2	1	0	208
bread, whole grain	1 slice (1 oz)	65	3	12	2	3	1	0	127
bread, whole wheat	1 slice (1 oz)	69	3	13	2	2	1	0	148
bun, hamburger	½ (1 oz)	60	3	11	1	2	1	1	110
bun, hot dog	½ (1 oz)	60	2	11	0	1	1	0	103
cornbread	1 oz	89	2	14	1	n/a	3	1	221
cracker, crispbread, rye	0.75 oz	78	2	17	4	0	0	0	56
cracker, graham	0.75 oz	89	1	16	1	7	2	0	127
cracker, graham, low-fat	0.75 oz	82	1	17	1	5	1	0	130

Food Item	Serving Size	Calories	Protein (g)	Carb (g)	Fiber (g)	Sugars (g)	Fat (g)	Sat Fat (g)	Sodium (mg)
cracker, matzo, plain	0.75 oz	84	2	18	1	0	0	0	0
cracker, saltine	0.75 oz	91	2	15	1	0	2	0	228
cracker, wheat	0.75 oz	94	2	15	2	0	4	1	140
croissant	½ medium	116	2	13	1	3	6	3	212
English muffin, whole wheat	½ (1 oz)	67	3	13	2	3	1	0	210
French toast	½ slice (1 oz)	74	3	8	0	n/a	4	1	156
muffin, blueberry	½ (1 oz)	79	2	14	1	6	2	0	127
muffin, bran	½ (1 oz)	107	2	14	1	13	5	1	98
pancake, buttermilk	1 (4") pancake (1 oz)	81	2	14	1	4	2	0	182
pancake, cornmeal	1 (4") pancake (1 oz)	43	1	7	0	1	1	0	52
phyllo dough	1 oz	85	2	15	1	0	2	0	137
taco shell, fried	1 (5") shell (0.5 oz)	50	1	7	0	0	2	1	45
tortilla, corn	1 (6") tortilla	57	1	12	2	0	1	0	12
tortilla, flour	1 (6") tortilla	100	3	16	1	1	2	1	204

Food Item	Serving Size	Calories	Protein (g)	Carb (g)	Fiber (g)	Sugars (g)	Fat (g)	Sat Fat (g)	Sodium (mg)
Breads and Crackers—*Continued*									
tortilla, wheat	1 (6") tortilla (1 oz)	73	3	20	2	n/a	0	0	171
waffle, plain	1 (1 oz)	84	2	13	1	1	3	0	193
Cereals									
All-Bran	⅓ cup	51	3	15	6	3	1	0	48
cereal, hot, multigrain	½ cup	101	3	20	2	1	1	0	1
Cheerios	½ cup	55	2	11	2	1	1	0	107
cornflakes	½ cup	51	1	12	0	1	0	0	101
Fiber One	½ cup	59	2	24	14	0	1	0	129
granola, low-fat, with raisins	½ cup	79	2	16	1	7	1	0	77
Kashi GoLean	½ cup	70	7	15	5	3	1	0	85
oat bran flakes	⅓ cup	55	2	12	2	3	0	0	6
oatmeal, old-fashioned, dry	¼ cup	74	3	14	2	0	2	0	1
raisin bran	⅓ cup	65	2	16	2	7	1	0	120
shredded wheat	1 single-serving box	85	3	21	3	0	0	0	2
Special K	½ cup	59	3	11	0	2	0	0	112

Food Item	Serving Size	Calories	Protein (g)	Carb (g)	Fiber (g)	Sugars (g)	Fat (g)	Sat Fat (g)	Sodium (mg)
Cheese									
American, pasteurized process, fat-free	1" cube	24	4	2	0	2	0	0	244
American, pasteurized process, low-fat	1" cube	32	4	1	0	0	1	1	251
Cheddar, fat-free	1" cube	40	8	1	0	1	0	0	220
Cheddar, low-fat	1" cube	30	4	0	0	0	1	1	106
cottage cheese, fat-free	4 oz	80	11	7	0	4	0	0	380
cottage cheese, 1% (low-fat), lactose-reduced	¼ cup	41	7	2	0	2	1	0	229
cream cheese, fat-free	2 Tbsp	28	4	2	0	0	0	0	158
cream cheese, low-fat	2 Tbsp	69	3	2	0	0	5	3	89
feta, low-fat	1¼" cube	50	6	1	0	0	3	2	370

Food Item	Serving Size	Calories	Protein (g)	Carb (g)	Fiber (g)	Sugars (g)	Fat (g)	Sat Fat (g)	Sodium (mg)
Cheese—*Continued*									
Laughing Cow, light, Swiss original	1 piece	35	2.5	1	0	1	2	1	260
Monterey Jack, low-fat	1" cube	53	5	0	0	0	4	2	96
mozzarella, part-skim	1" cube	53	5	1	0	0	4	2	93
mozzarella, string	1 stick	50	8	1	0	0	2	1	220
mozzarella, string, reduced-fat	1 stick	50	6	1	0	0	3	2	180
Parmesan, shredded	2 Tbsp	42	4	0	0	n/a	3	2	170
provolone	1" cube	60	4	0	0	0	5	3	149
ricotta, fat-free	¼ cup	50	5	5	0	2	0	0	65
ricotta, low-fat	¼ cup	86	7	3	0	0	5	3	78
Swiss, low-fat	1" cube	27	4	1	0	0	1	1	39
Condiments, Dressings, Marinades, Sandwich Toppings, and Spreads									
jam	1 Tbsp	56	0	14	0	10	0	0	6
jam, reduced-sugar	1 Tbsp	36	0	9	1	7	0	0	5
jelly	1 Tbsp	51	0	13	0	10	0	0	6

Food Item	Serving Size	Calories	Protein (g)	Carb (g)	Fiber (g)	Sugars (g)	Fat (g)	Sat Fat (g)	Sodium (mg)
jelly, reduced-sugar	1 Tbsp	34	0	9	0	9	0	0	0
ketchup	1 Tbsp	15	0	4	0	3	0	0	167
mayonnaise, fat-free	1 Tbsp	13	0	2	0	2	0	0	126
mayonnaise, light	1 Tbsp	46	0	1	0	1	5	1	95
mustard	1 Tbsp	10	1	1	0	0	0	0	168
olives, black	5 small	18	0	1	1	0	2	0	140
olives, green, pickled	5	41	0	1	1	0	4	1	441
pickle, dill	1 medium	12	0	3	1	2	0	0	833
pickles, bread-and-butter	¼ cup	34	0	8	1	4	0	0	286
pickle, sweet	1 medium	29	0	8	0	4	0	0	235
salsa	1 Tbsp	4	0	1	0	1	0	0	97
soy sauce	1 Tbsp	11	2	1	0	0	0	0	1,005
soy sauce, reduced-sodium	1 Tbsp	9	1	1	0	0	0	0	533
tahini	1 Tbsp	89	3	3	1	n/a	8	1	5
vinegar, balsamic	1 Tbsp	10	0	2	n/a	2	0	0	5
vinegar, white wine	1 Tbsp	5	0	2	0	0	0	0	0

Food Item	Serving Size	Calories	Protein (g)	Carb (g)	Fiber (g)	Sugars (g)	Fat (g)	Sat Fat (g)	Sodium (mg)
Dairy Products									
cream, light	1 Tbsp	29	0	1	0	0	3	2	6
sour cream, fat-free	1 Tbsp	10	0	2	0	0	0	0	20
sour cream, light	1 Tbsp	19	1	1	0	0	2	1	10
whipped topping, Cool Whip, fat-free	2 Tbsp	15	0	3	n/a	1	0	0	5
whipped topping, Cool Whip, light	2 Tbsp	20	0	3	n/a	1	1	1	0
yogurt, fruit, fat-free	4 oz	107	5	22	0	22	0	0	66
yogurt, plain	4 oz	69	4	5	0	5	4	2	52
yogurt, plain, fat-free	4 oz	50	5	9	0	6	0	0	67
yogurt, plain, low-fat	4 oz	80	7	10	0	9	1	1	95
Desserts and Frozen Treats									
frozen yogurt, chocolate	½ cup	110	3	19	1	18	3	2	55
frozen yogurt, chocolate, fat-free	½ cup	104	5	21	2	16	0	0	61

Food Item	Serving Size	Calories	Protein (g)	Carb (g)	Fiber (g)	Sugars (g)	Fat (g)	Sat Fat (g)	Sodium (mg)
frozen yogurt, vanilla	½ cup	140	3	21	0	16	5	3	45
frozen yogurt, vanilla, fat-free	½ cup	95	5	19	0	19	0	0	64
ice cream, chocolate, low-fat	½ cup	120	3	21	2	18	2	1	45
ice cream, vanilla, fat-free	½ cup	135	4	29	1	6	0	0	95
ice cream, vanilla, low-fat	½ cup	110	3	19	1	18	2	1	45
ice cream cone, sugar cone	½ cup	40	1	8	0	3	0	0	32
ice cream cone, wafer cone	½ cup	17	0	3	0	0	0	0	6
Fudgsicle, fat-free	1	70	3	14	1	10	0	0	50
Popsicle, cherry, sugar-free	1	15	0	4	0	0	0	0	0
sherbet, orange	½ cup	107	1	23	2	18	1	1	34
syrup, chocolate	1 Tbsp	50	1	12	n/a	10	0	0	13

Food Item	Serving Size	Calories	Protein (g)	Carb (g)	Fiber (g)	Sugars (g)	Fat (g)	Sat Fat (g)	Sodium (mg)
Eggs									
egg, hard-boiled	1 large	78	6	1	0	1	5	2	62
egg, poached	1 large	74	6	0	0	0	5	2	147
egg, scrambled	1 large	100	7	1	0	1	8	3	105
egg substitute, liquid	¼ cup	53	8	0	0	0	2	0	111
egg white, cooked	1 large	17	4	0	0	0	0	0	55
Fats and Oils									
butter, light, without salt	1 tsp	24	0	0	0	0	3	2	2
butter spread, Smart Balance 37% Light Buttery Spread	1 Tbsp	45	0	0	0	0	5	2	85
butter spread, Smart Balance 67% Buttery Spread	1 Tbsp	80	0	0	0	0	9	3	90
cooking spray	⅓ sec	0	0	0	0	0	0	0	0

Food Item	Serving Size	Calories	Protein (g)	Carb (g)	Fiber (g)	Sugars (g)	Fat (g)	Sat Fat (g)	Sodium (mg)
cooking spray, butter	1 sec	10	0	0	0	0	2	0	0
cooking spray, extra-virgin olive oil	½ sec	0	0	0	0	0	0	0	0
oil, almond	1 tsp	40	0	0	0	0	5	0	0
oil, canola	1 tsp	41	0	0	0	0	5	0	0
oil, flaxseed	1 tsp	40	0	0	0	0	5	0	0
oil, olive	1 tsp	40	0	0	0	0	5	1	0
oil, sesame	1 tsp	40	0	0	0	0	5	1	0
Fish									
anchovies, with oil, drained	3 oz	179	25	0	0	0	8	2	3,119
bass, sea, baked	3 oz	105	20	0	0	0	2	1	74
catfish, steamed	3 oz	144	17	0	0	0	8	2	51
cod, Atlantic, baked	3 oz	89	19	0	0	0	1	0	66
fish sticks	2 oz	112	4	13	1	2	4	n/a	n/a
fish tacos	4 oz	231	9	16	1	1	n/a	4	324
flounder, cooked	3 oz	101	19	0	0	0	2	0	101

Food Item	Serving Size	Calories	Protein (g)	Carb (g)	Fiber (g)	Sugars (g)	Fat (g)	Sat Fat (g)	Sodium (mg)
				Fish—*Continued*					
halibut, Atlantic, baked	3 oz	119	23	0	0	0	3	0	59
orange roughy, baked	3 oz	89	19	0	0	0	1	0	59
salmon, Alaskan chinook, canned	3 oz	226	26	0	0	0	n/a	n/a	n/a
salmon, Atlantic, wild, baked	3 oz	155	22	0	0	0	7	1	48
salmon, chinook, lox	3 oz	100	16	0	0	0	4	1	1,701
salmon, chinook, smoked	3 oz	100	16	0	0	0	4	1	667
swordfish, cooked	3 oz	122	16	0	0	0	6	2	101
tilapia, baked	3 oz	109	22	0	0	0	2	1	48
trout, rainbow, wild, baked	3 oz	128	19	0	0	0	5	1	48
tuna, chunk light, canned in water, drained	3 oz	105	23	0	0	0	0	0	345

Food Item	Serving Size	Calories	Protein (g)	Carb (g)	Fiber (g)	Sugars (g)	Fat (g)	Sat Fat (g)	Sodium (mg)
tuna, white, canned in water, drained	3 oz	109	20	0	0	0	3	1	321
tuna, yellowfin, baked	3 oz	118	25	0	0	0	1	0	40
Fresh and Dried Fruit									
apple	1	72	0	19	3	14	0	0	0
apricot	1	17	0	4	1	3	0	0	0
apricot, dried	1	18	0	4	0	n/a	0	0	0
avocado	¼ cup	58	1	3	2	0	5	1	3
banana	1 large (8")	121	1	31	4	17	0	0	1
blackberries	1 cup	62	2	14	7	6	1	0	1
blueberries	½ cup	41	1	11	2	7	0	0	1
cantaloupe, wedge	⅛ medium melon	23	1	6	n/a	n/a	0	0	11
cherries, sour	½ cup	39	1	9	1	7	0	0	2
cherries, sweet	½ cup	46	1	12	2	9	0	0	0
clementine	1	40	1	9	2	6	0	0	1
cranberries	1 cup	44	0	12	4	4	0	0	2
currants, red	½ cup	31	1	8	2	4	0	0	1
date, medjool, pitted	1	66	0	18	2	16	0	0	0

Food Item	Serving Size	Calories	Protein (g)	Carb (g)	Fiber (g)	Sugars (g)	Fat (g)	Sat Fat (g)	Sodium (mg)
Fresh and Dried Fruit—*Continued*									
fig	1 medium	37	0	10	1	8	0	0	1
fruit salad, canned, in water	½ cup	37	0	10	1	n/a	0	0	4
grapefruit	½ of medium	60	1	16	6	10	0	0	0
grapes, green	½ cup	55	1	14	1	12	0	0	2
grapes, red	½ cup	55	1	14	1	12	0	0	2
honeydew, balled	1 cup	64	1	16	1	14	0	0	32
lemon	1 medium	15	0	5	1	1	0	0	5
lime	1	20	0	7	2	1	0	0	1
mango	½	67	1	18	2	15	0	0	2
nectarine	1 medium	70	1	17	1	13	0	0	0
orange	1 small (2⅜")	45	1	11	2	9	0	0	0
orange, blood	1 medium	70	1	16	3	12	0	0	0
papaya	1 small	59	1	15	3	9	0	0	5
passion fruit, purple	1	17	0	4	2	2	0	0	5
peach	1 medium	38	1	9	1	8	0	0	0

Food Item	Serving Size	Calories	Protein (g)	Carb (g)	Fiber (g)	Sugars (g)	Fat (g)	Sat Fat (g)	Sodium (mg)
pear	½	50	1	13	2	9	1	0	0
pineapple, diced	½ cup	37	0	10	1	7	0	0	1
plantain, cooked, mashed	¼ cup	58	0	16	1	7	0	0	3
plum	1 (2⅛")	30	0	8	1	7	0	0	0
pomegranate	½ of 3⅜"	53	0	13	0	13	0	0	2
prunes	3 medium	50	1	13	2	6	0	0	3
raisins, golden, seedless, packed	2 Tbsp	65	1	16	1	15	0	0	5
raisins, purple, seedless, packed	2 Tbsp	61	1	16	1	n/a	0	0	6
raspberries, black	3 oz	61	1	14	1	4	0	0	0
raspberries, red	3 oz	44	1	10	6	4	1	0	1
rhubarb	1 stalk	11	0	2	1	1	0	0	2
strawberry	1 medium	4	0	1	0	1	0	0	0
tangelo, Minneola	1	70	1	13	2	11	1	0	0
tangerine	1 medium	50	1	13	3	8	1	0	0

Food Item	Serving Size	Calories	Protein (g)	Carb (g)	Fiber (g)	Sugars (g)	Fat (g)	Sat Fat (g)	Sodium (mg)
Grains and Rice									
barley, pearled, cooked	¼ cup	48	1	11	1	0	0	0	1
barley, whole, cooked	¼ cup	68	2	15	2	n/a	1	0	0
buckwheat groats (kasha), roasted, cooked	⅓ cup	51	2	11	2	1	0	0	2
bulgur, cooked	⅓ cup	50	2	11	3	0	0	0	3
corn flour, whole grain, yellow	2 Tbsp	53	1	11	2	0	1	0	1
couscous, cooked	⅓ cup	59	2	12	1	0	0	0	3
hominy, cooked	½ cup	69	1	12	2	n/a	1	0	173
millet, cooked	¼ cup	52	2	10	1	0	0	0	1
oat bran, cooked	⅓ cup	29	2	8	2	n/a	1	0	1
oats, unprocessed whole grain	2 Tbsp	76	3	13	2	n/a	1	0	0
quinoa, cooked	¼ cup	81	3	15	1	n/a	1	0	4

Food Item	Serving Size	Calories	Protein (g)	Carb (g)	Fiber (g)	Sugars (g)	Fat (g)	Sat Fat (g)	Sodium (mg)
rice, brown, long-grain, cooked	¼ cup	54	1	11	1	0	0	0	2
rice, white, short-grain, cooked	¼ cup	60	1	12	0	n/a	0	0	0
risotto, rice, Arborio, dry	2 Tbsp	85	2	19	1	0	0	0	0
semolina, unenriched	2 Tbsp	75	3	15	1	0	0	0	0
wheat flour, whole grain	2 Tbsp	51	2	11	2	0	0	0	1
wheat, sprouted	2 Tbsp	27	1	6	0	0	0	2	n/a
Meats: Beef									
bottom round, all lean, cooked	3 oz	139	24	0	0	0	5	2	31
brisket, flat, lean, braised	3 oz	174	28	0	0	0	6	2	46
chuck roast, lean, braised	3 oz	179	28	0	0	0	6	2	56
corned beef, cooked	3 oz	213	15	0	0	0	16	5	964
filet mignon, lean, broiled	3 oz	179	24	0	0	0	9	3	54
flank steak, lean, broiled	3 oz	158	24	0	0	0	6	3	48

Food Item	Serving Size	Calories	Protein (g)	Carb (g)	Fiber (g)	Sugars (g)	Fat (g)	Sat Fat (g)	Sodium (mg)
Meats: Beef—*Continued*									
ground beef, 80% lean, pan-broiled	3 oz	230	22	0	0	0	15	6	64
hot dog, beef, 97% fat-free	1.7 oz	45	6	3	0	0	1	1	400
pastrami, beef, 98% fat-free	1 oz	27	6	0	0	0	0	0	286
rib steak, select lean, with bone, roasted	3 oz	81	11	0	0	0	4	2	28
salami, beef, cooked	1 oz	73	4	1	0	0	0	6	3
sausage, beef, precooked	1 oz	115	4	0	0	0	11	4	258
short ribs, lean, with bone, braised	3 oz	65	7	0	0	0	4	2	13
steak, sirloin strip, ⅛ trim, broiled	3 oz	236	22	0	0	0	16	6	44
tenderloin, select lean, boneless, roasted	3 oz	152	24	0	0	0	6	2	50

Food Item	Serving Size	Calories	Protein (g)	Carb (g)	Fiber (g)	Sugars (g)	Fat (g)	Sat Fat (g)	Sodium (mg)
Meats: Lamb									
ground lamb, 20% fat, broiled	3 oz	241	21	0	0	0	17	7	69
kebab, lean, braised	3 oz	190	29	0	0	0	7	3	60
leg, Australian, whole, lean, roasted	3 oz	162	23	0	0	0	7	3	61
sirloin chop, Australian, lean, broiled	3 oz	160	24	0	0	0	7	3	56
Meats: Pork									
bacon, Canadian, grilled	1 oz	52	7	0	0	0	2	1	439
bacon, medium slice, cooked	0.2 oz	34	2	0	0	0	3	1	146
chop, center lean, with bone, braised	2.6 oz	149	22	0	0	0	6	2	46
ground pork, cooked	3 oz	253	22	0	0	0	18	7	62
ham, low-sodium, 96% fat-free	1 oz	31	5	1	0	1	1	0	235
hot dog, pork	2.7 oz	204	10	0	0	0	18	7	620

Food Item	Serving Size	Calories	Protein (g)	Carb (g)	Fiber (g)	Sugars (g)	Fat (g)	Sat Fat (g)	Sodium (mg)
Meats: Pork—Continued									
hot dog, pork, beef, and turkey, fat-free	1.8 oz	50	6	6	0	2	0	0	490
prosciutto, sliced	0.5 oz	50	4	0	0	0	2	1	375
ribs, country-style, lean, braised	3 oz	199	22	0	0	0	12	4	54
sausage, pork, frozen	1 oz	65	4	0	0	0	5	1	144
tenderloin, roasted	3 oz	139	24	0	0	0	4	1	48
Meats: Veal									
breast, braised	3 oz	226	23	0	0	0	14	6	55
ground veal, 8% fat, broiled	3 oz	146	21	0	0	0	6	3	71
liver, braised	3 oz	163	24	3	0	0	5	2	66
loin chop cutlet, braised	3 oz	242	26	0	0	0	15	6	68
shank roast, braised	3 oz	151	27	0	0	0	4	1	80

Food Item	Serving Size	Calories	Protein (g)	Carb (g)	Fiber (g)	Sugars (g)	Fat (g)	Sat Fat (g)	Sodium (mg)
Nuts, Seeds, and Nut Butters									
almond butter, plain, with salt	1 Tbsp	99	2	3	1	1	9	1	70
almonds, dry-roasted, without salt	1 Tbsp	51	2	2	1	0	5	0	0
cashew butter, organic	1 Tbsp	83	3	6	1	n/a	6	1	0
cashews, dry-roasted, without salt	1 Tbsp	49	1	3	0	0	4	1	1
chestnuts, European, roasted	1 Tbsp	22	0	5	0	1	0	0	0
coconut, dried, shredded, unsweetened	1 Tbsp	18	0	1	0	0	3	1	1
flaxseeds	1 Tbsp	45	1	1	1	0	4	0	0
hazelnuts (filberts), blanched	0.5 oz	89	2	2	2	0	9	1	0
peanut butter, natural	1 Tbsp	100	4	4	1	1	8	1	60

Food Item	Serving Size	Calories	Protein (g)	Carb (g)	Fiber (g)	Sugars (g)	Fat (g)	Sat Fat (g)	Sodium (mg)
Nuts, Seeds, and Nut Butters—*Continued*									
peanut butter, reduced-fat	1 Tbsp	81	4	5	1	2	5	1	89
peanuts, dry-roasted, without salt	1 Tbsp	53	2	2	1	0	5	1	1
pecans, raw, halved	1 Tbsp	48	1	1	0	0	5	0	0
pine nuts (pignoli), dried	1 Tbsp	57	1	1	0	0	6	0	0
pistachios, dry-roasted, without salt	1 Tbsp	46	2	2	1	1	4	0	1
pumpkin and squash seed kernels, roasted, without salt	1 oz	147	9	4	1	0	12	2	5
sesame seeds, dried, whole	1 Tbsp	52	2	2	1	0	4	1	1
sunflower seeds, dry-roasted, without salt	1 Tbsp	47	2	3	1	0	4	0	0
walnuts, English, dried, halved	1 Tbsp	41	1	1	0	0	4	0	0

Food Item	Serving Size	Calories	Protein (g)	Carb (g)	Fiber (g)	Sugars (g)	Fat (g)	Sat Fat (g)	Sodium (mg)
Poultry: Chicken									
breast, boneless, without skin, raw	4 oz	132	25	0	0	0	3	1	55
breast, fat-free, oven-roasted, sliced	3 oz	67	14	2	0	0	0	0	924
drumstick, without skin, cooked	3 oz	146	24	0	0	0	5	1	91
ground chicken, raw	4 oz	150	18	0	0	0	9	3	65
Poultry: Turkey									
breast, tenderloin, raw	4 oz	120	28	0	0	0	2	0	65
burger, Jennie-O Turkey Store Lean Turkey Burger Patties	112 g	160	23	0	0	0	8	2.5	80
dark meat, without skin, raw	4 oz	142	23	0	0	0	5	2	87

Food Item	Serving Size	Calories	Protein (g)	Carb (g)	Fiber (g)	Sugars (g)	Fat (g)	Sat Fat (g)	Sodium (mg)
Poultry: Turkey—Continued									
ground turkey, Jennie-O Turkey Store Lean	112 g	160	23	0	0	0	8	2.5	80
light meat, without skin, roasted	3 oz	134	25	0	0	3	1	0	54
light meat, with skin, roasted	3 oz	168	24	0	0	0	7	2	54
meatball, turkey	1 oz	48	6	2	0	0	2	1	36
meat loaf, turkey	4 oz slice	184	22	8	1	n/a	7	2	139
sausage, Jennie-O Turkey Store Breakfast Sausage Links	56 g	140	9	0	0	0	11	3	360
Seafood									
crab, blue, flaked, steamed	3 oz	87	17	0	0	0	2	0	237
crab leg, Alaskan king, steamed	3 oz	83	16	0	0	0	1	0	912

Food Item	Serving Size	Calories	Protein (g)	Carb (g)	Fiber (g)	Sugars (g)	Fat (g)	Sat Fat (g)	Sodium (mg)
lobster, baked, diced	3 oz	99	17	1	0	0	3	1	335
shrimp, raw	1 medium	6	1	0	0	0	0	0	9
shrimp, sautéed	3 oz	132	21	1	0	n/a	4	1	183
shrimp, steamed	1 large	5	1	0	0	0	0	0	12
Soups, Sauces, and Gravies									
broth, beef, low-sodium	1 cup	38	5	1	0	1	1	0	72
broth, beef, 93% fat-free	1 cup	15	3	0	0	0	0	0	450
broth, chicken, fat-free	1 cup	25	6	0	0	0	0	0	390
broth, chicken, low-sodium	1 cup	38	5	3	0	0	1	0	72
chowder, clam, Manhattan-style	1 cup	78	2	12	1	1	2	0	578
chowder, clam, New England–style	1 cup	190	6	20	1	3	10	3	920
sauce, taco, green	1 Tbsp	5	0	1	0	0	0	0	96

Food Item	Serving Size	Calories	Protein (g)	Carb (g)	Fiber (g)	Sugars (g)	Fat (g)	Sat Fat (g)	Sodium (mg)
Soups, Sauces, and Gravies—*Continued*									
sauce, tomato, with salt	½ cup	39	2	9	2	5	0	0	642
soup, beef barley	1 cup	90	7	15	0	0	1	0	970
soup, beef vegetable	1 cup	120	9	17	n/a	n/a	2	1	1,259
soup, black bean, low-fat, organic	½ cup	70	4	13	3	4	1	0	290
soup, chicken noodle, low-sodium	1 cup	76	4	11	1	0	2	1	426
soup, chicken rice, low-fat	1 cup	130	8	21	2	4	2	0	390
soup, chicken vegetable, low-sodium	1 cup	166	12	19	1	2	5	1	84
soup, cream of celery, 98% fat-free	½ cup	60	1	8	1	1	3	1	780
soup, cream of chicken, reduced-sodium	1 cup	66	2	11	0	0	2	1	405

Food Item	Serving Size	Calories	Protein (g)	Carb (g)	Fiber (g)	Sugars (g)	Fat (g)	Sat Fat (g)	Sodium (mg)
soup, cream of potato	1 cup	68	2	11	0	n/a	2	1	930
soup, French onion	1 cup	43	2	6	1	4	1	0	856
soup, lentil, fat-free	½ cup	55	5	13	5	3	0	0	225
soup, minestrone	1 cup	120	5	22	4	4	2	0	1,050
soup, miso with tofu	1 cup	220	10	42	0	2	2	0	1,380
soup, split pea, fat-free, organic	½ cup	50	4	10	2	2	0	0	285
soup, tomato	1 cup	161	6	22	3	15	6	3	744
soup, vegetable	1 cup	70	3	8	1	1	3	1	889
soup, vegetable chicken	1 cup	50	3	8	n/a	n/a	1	0	807
Soy Foods									
cheese, soy	1 oz	8	1	1	n/a	n/a	0	n/a	n/a
miso	1 Tbsp	34	2	5	1	1	1	0	640
tempeh, three-grain	4 oz	190	12	25	6	2	4	2	17
tofu, silken, firm	4 oz	70	8	3	0	3	3	0	41

Food Item	Serving Size	Calories	Protein (g)	Carb (g)	Fiber (g)	Sugars (g)	Fat (g)	Sat Fat (g)	Sodium (mg)
Soy Foods—Continued									
tofu, silken, soft	4 oz	63	5	3	0	1	3	0	6
yogurt, tofu	4 oz	123	5	21	0	2	2	0	46
Sweeteners									
agave nectar	1 tsp	15	0	4	0	4	0	0	4
honey	1 tsp	21	0	6	0	0	0	0	0
maple syrup	1 tsp	17	0	4	0	4	0	0	1
molasses, blackstrap	1 tsp	16	0	4	0	3	0	0	4
molasses, dark	1 tsp	17	0	5	0	5	0	0	1
stevia	1 packet	4	0	1	0	0	0	0	0
sugar, brown, unpacked	1 tsp	11	0	3	0	3	0	0	1
sugar, cane, organic, unrefined	1 tsp	16	0	4	0	4	0	0	0
sugar, white	1 tsp	16	0	4	0	4	0	0	0
Vegetables									
artichoke	1 medium	60	4	13	7	3	0	0	120
artichoke hearts, cooked, with salt, drained	½ cup	42	3	9	5	1	0	0	278

Food Item	Serving Size	Calories	Protein (g)	Carb (g)	Fiber (g)	Sugars (g)	Fat (g)	Sat Fat (g)	Sodium (mg)
arugula (rocket)	4 oz	28	3	4	2	2	1	0	31
asparagus, cooked	4 oz	25	3	5	2	1	0	0	4
beets, cooked, without salt	½ cup	37	1	8	2	7	0	0	65
bell pepper, chopped	1 cup	39	1	9	3	4	0	0	3
broccoli florets	1 cup	20	2	4	2	0	0	0	19
brussels sprouts	1 cup	38	3	8	3	2	0	0	22
cabbage, shredded	1 cup	17	1	4	2	2	0	0	13
carrot	1 medium	25	1	6	2	3	0	0	42
carrot, baby	1 medium	4	0	1	1	1	0	0	8
cauliflower	¼ medium head	36	3	8	4	4	0	0	43
celery	1 medium stalk	9	0	2	1	1	0	0	50
collard greens, chopped	1 cup	11	1	2	1	0	0	0	7
corn, sweet white	1 small ear	63	2	14	2	2	1	0	11
corn, sweet yellow	½ cup	66	2	15	2	2	1	0	12

Food Item	Serving Size	Calories	Protein (g)	Carb (g)	Fiber (g)	Sugars (g)	Fat (g)	Sat Fat (g)	Sodium (mg)
				Vegetables—*Continued*					
cucumber	1 (8")	45	2	11	2	5	0	0	6
eggplant, cubed, cooked, with salt, drained	1 cup	35	1	9	2	3	0	0	237
endive	½ head	44	3	9	8	1	1	0	56
fennel bulb, sliced	1 cup	27	1	7	3	0	0	0	45
garlic	1 clove	4	0	1	0	0	0	0	0
green beans	1 cup	38	2	8	3	2	0	0	2
jicama (yam bean), chopped	½ cup	25	0	6	3	1	0	0	3
kale, Scotch, chopped	1 cup	28	2	6	1	1	0	0	47
leeks, sliced	10 slices	37	1	8	1	2	0	0	12
lettuce, Bibb	4 medium leaves	5	1	1	0	0	0	0	2
lettuce, iceberg	5 large leaves	10	1	2	1	1	0	0	8
mushrooms, cremini	5	15	2	3	0	1	0	0	4
mushrooms, portobello	2 oz	15	1	3	1	1	0	0	3
mushrooms, shiitake, dried	1 Tbsp	30	2	5	1	n/a	0	0	8

Food Item	Serving Size	Calories	Protein (g)	Carb (g)	Fiber (g)	Sugars (g)	Fat (g)	Sat Fat (g)	Sodium (mg)
okra, cooked	1 cup	52	4	11	5	5	1	0	6
onion, red, sliced	1 large slice	16	0	4	1	2	0	0	1
onion, yellow, chopped	½ cup	34	1	8	1	3	0	0	2
palm, hearts	1 oz	33	1	7	1	5	0	0	4
parsnips, sliced	½ cup	49	1	12	3	3	0	0	7
peas, green, cooked	½ cup	62	4	11	4	4	0	0	3
peas, snow	½ cup	13	1	2	1	1	0	0	1
pepper, hot chile, green	1	18	1	4	1	2	0	0	3
pepper, hot chile, red	1	18	1	4	1	2	0	0	4
potato, baked, with skin	1 medium	162	4	36	4	3	0	0	12
pumpkin, canned, without salt	½ cup	42	1	10	4	4	0	0	6
pumpkin, cubed	½ cup	15	1	4	0	1	0	0	1
radicchio	10 leaves	18	1	4	1	0	0	0	18
radish, red, sliced	½ cup	9	0	2	1	1	0	0	23

Food Item	Serving Size	Calories	Protein (g)	Carb (g)	Fiber (g)	Sugars (g)	Fat (g)	Sat Fat (g)	Sodium (mg)
			Vegetables—*Continued*						
rutabaga	1 medium	139	5	31	10	22	1	0	77
shallots, chopped	¼ cup	29	1	7	0	1	0	0	5
spinach	3 oz	20	2	3	2	0	0	0	67
squash, butternut, cubed	½ cup	54	1	14	2	3	0	0	5
squash, spaghetti, baked	1 cup	42	1	10	2	4	0	0	28
squash, summer	1 medium	31	2	7	2	4	0	0	4
squash, winter acorn, cubed	½ cup	28	1	7	1	2	0	0	2
sweet potato, baked, with skin	1 small	95	2	22	3	16	0	0	10
tomatillo, chopped	½ cup	21	1	4	1	3	1	0	1
tomato paste, without salt	1 Tbsp	13	1	3	1	2	0	0	16
tomato, red, canned	4 oz	19	1	4	1	3	0	0	145
turnip, cubed	1 cup	36	8	2	5	0	0	0	87

Food Item	Serving Size	Calories	Protein (g)	Carb (g)	Fiber (g)	Sugars (g)	Fat (g)	Sat Fat (g)	Sodium (mg)
water chestnuts, canned	1 oz	14	0	3	3	1	0	0	3
watercress, chopped	1 cup	4	1	0	0	0	0	0	14
yam, cooked, without salt	¼ cup	39	1	9	1	0	0	0	3
zucchini	1 medium	35	2	7	2	3	0	0	20
Vegetarian Protein									
breakfast link, soy	0.9 oz	30	6	2	1	1	0	0	195
burger, MorningStar Farms Garden Veggie Patties	1 patty	119	11	10	4	1	4	1	382
burger, soy	2.5 oz	125	13	9	3	1	4	1	385
hot dog, MorningStar Farms America's Original Veggie Dog	1	112	10	4	3	1	6	1	431
soy, ground, Melissa's	2 oz	70	11	4	3	0	3	0	250

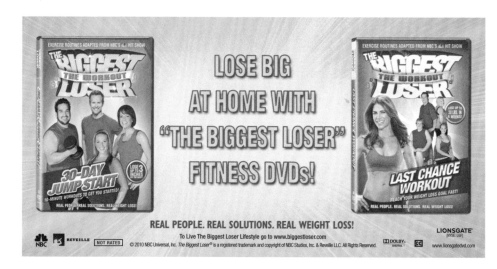
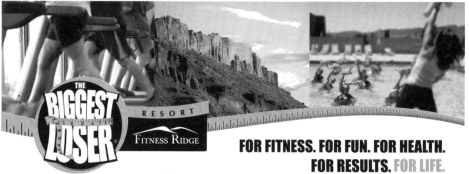

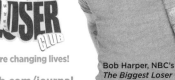
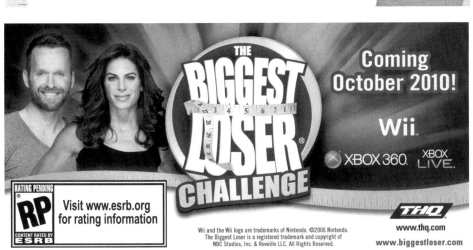

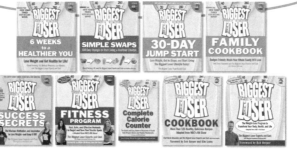
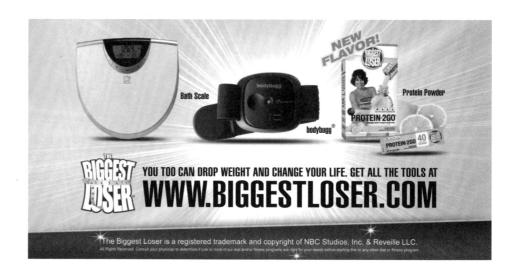